COMMUNITY-BASED
HEALTH
INTERVENTIONS

COMMUNITY-BASED HEALTH INTERVENTIONS

Principles and Applications

SALLY GUTTMACHER

PATRICIA J. KELLY

YUMARY RUIZ-JANECKO

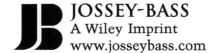

JOSSEY-BASS
A Wiley Imprint
www.josseybass.com

Published by Jossey-Bass
A Wiley Imprint
989 Market Street, San Francisco, CA 94103-1741—www.josseybass.com

Readers should be aware that Internet Web sites offered as citations and/or sources for further information may have changed or disappeared between the time this was written and when it is read.

Limit of Liability/Disclaimer of Warranty: While the publisher and author have used their best efforts in preparing this book, they make no representations or warranties with respect to the accuracy or completeness of the contents of this book and specifically disclaim any implied warranties of merchantability or fitness for a particular purpose. No warranty may be created or extended by sales representatives or written sales materials. The advice and strategies contained herein may not be suitable for your situation. You should consult with a professional where appropriate. Neither the publisher nor author shall be liable for any loss of profit or any other commercial damages, including but not limited to special, incidental, consequential, or other damages.

Jossey-Bass books and products are available through most bookstores. To contact Jossey-Bass directly call our Customer Care Department within the U.S. at 800-956-7739, outside the U.S. at 317-572-3986, or fax 317-572-4002.

Jossey-Bass also publishes its books in a variety of electronic formats. Some content that appears in print may not be available in electronic books.

Library of Congress Cataloging-in-Publication Data
Guttmacher, Sally.
    Community-based health interventions : principles and applications / Sally Guttmacher, Patricia J. Kelly, Yumary Ruiz-Janecko.—1st ed.
        p. ; cm.
    Includes bibliographical references and index.
    ISBN 978-0-7879-8311-6 (pbk.)
        1. Primary health care.   2. Community health services—United States.   I. Kelly, Patricia J. (Patricia Jane)   II. Ruiz-Janecko, Yumary, 1969-   III. Title.   [DNLM: 1. Health Promotion—methods.   2. Community Health Services. WA 590 G985c 2010]
    RA427.9.G88 2010
    362.12—dc22
                                                                                2009041344

FIRST EDITION

PB Printing   10 9 8 7 6 5 4 3 2

CONTENTS

PART ONE
INTRODUCING COMMUNITY-BASED
INTERVENTIONS   1

TABLES, FIGURE, AND EXHIBIT

TABLES

FIGURE

EXHIBIT

PREFACE

As instructors to students who ventured into the community, we could not find a text that covered the entire process of doing a community-based health intervention. This book is designed for these students and practitioners who are untrained in conducting such fieldwork. This book will review the skills necessary to implement a community-based health intervention to change health in a community setting. Community-based health interventions (referred to below and in future chapters as community interventions) differ from those undertaken by health care providers in the clinical setting, which involve a one-on-one interaction. Health interventions in a community setting involve groups of individuals and take place in any of the diverse venues that make up community—schools, churches, libraries, community centers, and public health departments with Women, Infants, and Children (WIC) programs. Community-based health interventions are important because they aim both to reduce the impact of disease, health-related conditions like obesity, and health-related risk taking such as cigarette smoking and to create a supportive environment for the maintenance of the behavior changes. To implement such interventions does not require a medical background; however, a specific set of skills is needed. To successfully implement community interventions, practitioners and researchers must have good communication skills, especially with people who come from backgrounds different from their own. They must feel comfortable talking to groups. Most important, practitioners and researchers should be able to think on their feet—that is, to be able to make decisions and keep an intervention going in an environment that may have limited resources and is complex and often unfamiliar. Such an environment differs from that of a clinic or hospital, which has clearly defined resources present in very controlled settings. This difference in environments can make clinicians uncomfortable at first, but is less problematic for public health practitioners if they have never been exposed to a clinical environment and do not have to make the transition from a patient or client focus to targeting a group or community. The frequent surprises and adaptations that come with working in community settings provide a rich sense of satisfaction and connection to those willing to engage in this work. We wrote this book because we have participated in a variety of community-level health interventions and have experienced such satisfaction. We hope to pass on to students the skills and the satisfaction that we have been privileged to experience in our work.

This book is intended as an introduction to the field of community-based health interventions and is not meant to be a comprehensive manual of all nuances and facets of developing interventions. The chapters review and summarize topics that could each easily be a book in itself. Students and practitioners who are not experienced in community work can progress through the various steps necessary to acquire the skills to complete, evaluate, disseminate, and sustain a community-based health intervention.

The text is set within the context of ecological theory. This theory posits an approach to health problems at different social levels starting with a group, moving to the organizational level, and finally to a policy level, where the entire community may be involved. This theory is used by public health practitioners and clearly distinguishes health programs taking place at the community level from those implemented at the clinical or individual level. The text will provide examples of community-based health interventions at each of the four ecological levels. The group level focuses on individuals who share a health risk or some other characteristic. The organization level includes interventions that take place throughout an individual school or all the schools in a district. For students using this book, interventions at the group or organizational level will probably be most appropriate. Community-level interventions work to change the total environmental or social structure of a geographic community, usually through a social marketing campaign. Policy-level interventions are the fourth ecological level and include changes in laws or regulations such as communitywide no-smoking policies.

The book is organized into four sections. The first section provides background information about why interventions in communities are important, the history of several major community interventions, ethical issues important to keep in mind during the design and implementation of interventions, and the different types of interventions that might be implemented. The second section covers the thinking and activities that must be completed to develop an intervention and helps students understand the theoretical basis of their intervention and how data will be managed. The third section projects the student into the field, assessing the needs and strengths of a particular community, gaining community support, defining the goals of an intervention, and actually getting started. This section also contains information on obtaining material and financial support and on strategies for continuing the intervention beyond its initial phase. The final section examines current work and problems encountered, as well as projecting how the field may change and expand in the near future. Each chapter of the book contains a number of practice exercises or activities to help students develop the skills they will need as practitioners. We hope these exercises will prove useful to students in the many professions that develop interventions at the population or community level, such as public health, social work, and nursing. Discussion issues are also raised at the end of each chapter. Additional readings and references are provided at the end of each chapter so that students who are interested in the particular areas covered can explore them in greater depth. Finally, the book contains a glossary defining words or phrases that may be unfamiliar to students who are just being introduced to the field.

ACKNOWLEDGMENTS

We have many people to thank, starting with the students we have taught, including graduate students Amarilis Cespedes, Jaugha Nielsen-Bobbit, and Jennifer Mills, who helped us by critically reading the text. We would also like to thank Benjamin Alan Holtzman for providing us a window into the future. We could not have written this book without our very supportive partners, William R. Breen, Joshua Freeman, and Gerald Andrew Janecko, who willingly held down the forts when we took off without them for a book-writing retreat in Tucson.

THE AUTHORS

Sally Guttmacher, PhD, is professor of public health at New York University, where she directs the MPH Program in Community Public Health. She is also a Visiting Professor in Public Health at the University of Cape Town. Her doctorate in sociomedical sciences is from Columbia University. She has been involved in community-based health interventions and evaluation research in New York City and in Cape Town, South Africa, and is coauthor of the book *Community-Based Health Organizations* (Jossey-Bass, 2005). She has been the president of the Public Health Association of New York City, the chair of the Medical Care Section of the American Public Health Association, the chair of the Council of Public Health Programs, and is on the National Board of Public Health Examiners. Her recent research interests include program evaluation, the prevention and treatment of HIV/AIDS, and the reduction of sexual risk behavior in refugee populations.

Patricia J. Kelly, PhD, MPH, APRN, is professor at the University of Missouri-Kansas City, School of Nursing. Her PhD in Public Health is from the University of Illinois at Chicago. Her clinical and research work has focused on improving the conditions of health for women and children in underserved populations. Kelly has conducted a number of NIH-, state-, and foundation-funded community-based research studies in Hispanic and African American communities. Her work has focused on reproductive health and violence prevention and has used a variety of research and evaluation methodologies, including community-based participatory action research.

Yumary Ruiz-Janecko is clinical assistant professor of public health and the Public Health Internship Director in the Department of Nutrition, Food Studies, and Public Health at New York University (NYU). She earned her PhD in health promotion and disease prevention, with a focus on health policy and health advocacy, from Purdue University in 2006. Her research interests include the links between migration and health and the impact of empowerment on health outcomes at individual, community, and system levels. Her current research focuses on examining HIV risk behaviors among recent Mexican immigrants residing in New York City. Prior to joining NYU, her research investigated the use of the Internet by nonprofit organizations, specifically advocacy organizations, and its association to sociopolitical empowerment. She has taught and developed numerous graduate and undergraduate courses, and as a public health practitioner she has coordinated and implemented health programs using multicomponent, multisectoral, and multisetting approaches.

Diana Silver, PhD, MPH, is an assistant professor of public health at the New York University's Steinhardt School of Culture, Education and Human Development. She has been working in the field of public health for more than two decades. Silver's research explores the ways in which local government policies and programs can be used to more effectively address those needs. She began her career focused on the developing policies and programs that could address the epidemics of AIDS, substance abuse, and violence in New York City in such settings as schools, workplaces, jails, and through community-based organizations. For the past decade, she served as the project director of the national evaluation of the Robert Wood Johnson Foundation's Urban Health Initiative, which aimed to improve health and safety outcomes for children and youth in some of America's most distressed cities.

COMMUNITY-BASED HEALTH INTERVENTIONS

PART

1

INTRODUCING COMMUNITY-BASED INTERVENTIONS

CHAPTER

1

IMPROVING HEALTH IN COMMUNITY SETTINGS

LEARNING OBJECTIVES

- Explain the components of an ecological approach to health
- Distinguish an ecological from an individual approach to health interventions
- Recognize different ways in which community can be defined

OVERVIEW

Ecological theory provides an overview to understanding interventions that take place in community settings. This chapter will explain the differences between interventions taking place in community settings and those taking place in clinical settings. Examples of community interventions will be provided.

DEFINING COMMUNITY

A **community** is a group of people connected by visible and invisible links. Communities are defined in different ways. *Geographic communities* have geographic, physical, or political boundaries, whereas *communities of interest* are connected not by physical space but by the sharing of an interest, behavior, risk, or characteristic, and *professional communities* share knowledge and skills as well as interests.

Place Can Define a Community

Geographic communities can have political boundaries such as municipal lines that may be more or less arbitrary, but provide residents with a sense of identity that is generally distinct from the adjacent area—such as Center City, as opposed to South Center City. Geographic communities can also be defined by geographic or physical boundaries that unite people inside the boundaries (north of the river) or make them distinct and separate from adjacent groups (the other side of the railroad tracks). The use of geographic features to define communities is necessary for the work of policy makers and planners who use, for example, census tracks, health districts, or hospital catchment areas for planning purposes. While these boundaries may or may not indicate differences between people who live in these areas, they provide a useful delineation in which to conduct interventions.

Communities Defined by a Shared Concern

Communities of shared concerns or interest can be linked by something as inherent as racial, ethnic, or national background and the history, values, culture, and customs that are part of that background. The social units that structure people's work, school, or other daily activities provide another form of community. These units can generally be broken down further by age (third-grade class as distinct from the sixth-grade class in a suburban elementary school), by role (nurses as distinct from physicians in a public hospital), or by status (students as distinct from teachers in the suburban elementary school; patients as distinct from providers in the hospital). An important community of shared interest for students and practitioners concerned with health issues is the groups of people with potential, current, or past shared disease and behavior or health risk. Women with a positive BRCA gene (indicating a higher-than-average risk for breast cancer), women receiving radiation treatment for breast cancer (current disease), and women in a cancer survivors support group (past disease) are all part of a potential or real community of interest.

The definition of community is important for public health practitioners because health interventions must target a specific community. How a **target community** is defined determines how resources will be allocated, how an intervention will be delivered, and how a message will be framed.

An example of the importance of defining a target community can be seen in designing a smoking cessation intervention. If the target audience is undergraduate students, focusing on the long-term health effects of tobacco use is unlikely to be an effective strategy because this population is in an adolescent phase of development, believing that "it won't happen to me" and focusing on today rather than the future. A more successful strategy for smoking cessation with this population would be an intervention demonstrating ways to resist social pressures while gaining peer acceptance. If the target population of a smoking cessation intervention is pregnant women, however, a message about the impact of cigarette smoking on healthy pregnancy outcomes will be more effective than one that stresses prevention of lung cancer and chronic obstructive pulmonary disease.

Demographic variables such as race, ethnicity, education level, age, gender, and class describe both geographic and common-interest communities. Many interventions will have a target community arising from more than one of these variables. A breast cancer survivor group for women in their sixties will have different issues from women in their thirties; an intervention to increase mammogram screening among African American women will need to incorporate different cultural strategies from one aimed at Latinas. Educational messages on mammogram screening for middle-class women with private health insurance may differ from messages with the same goal designed for women relying on public hospitals and clinics. Knowledge of the cultural background, health beliefs, developmental stage, socioeconomic status, and literacy levels must all be incorporated into the content of any health intervention.

ECOLOGICAL THEORY AND LEVELS OF PREVENTION

Ecological theory postulates health to be the result of a dynamic interplay between demographic variables and the physical and social environment. It expands on the model of living organisms as self-regulating systems by including the families, organizations, and communities in which we interact on a daily basis; a disturbance in any part of the system has an effect on the other parts (Bronfenbrenner, 1979). Individuals, families, and communities are not isolated entities, but rather an interrelated ecological system with each adapting to changes that occur in other parts of the organization. Each component of the system participates in determining health. Key factors in ecological theory that have a disproportionate influence on health include socioeconomic status, family, work (for adults), and school (for children) (Grzywacz & Fuqua, 2000). Consideration and integration of one or more of these factors cannot be considered in isolation from the others.

Ecological Theory Applied to Community-Based Intervention

Applying ecological theory to community-based health interventions requires an understanding of these three principles:

■   Health is the result of a fit between individuals and their environment

■   Environmental and social conditions interact with an individual to exert an important influence on health

■   A multidisciplinary approach to health is necessary (Grzywacz & Fuqua, 2000)

This appreciation of health as influenced by other than individual behavior has important implications for health promotion interventions. **Community-based health interventions** move beyond a focus on changing the behavior of individuals and instead acknowledge the importance of interpersonal or group behavior, institutional climate, community resources, and policy effects. Community-based interventions therefore work with groups such as women over age fifty in a church, institutions such as all teachers in a district's school system, communities with geographic or political boundaries, and large populations covered by specific policies.

Prevention Efforts Focused on the Community

The influence of social and environmental factors on health behaviors and outcomes occurred around the same time as an understanding of the limitations of the individualistic medical model in changing health behaviors and outcomes. While health care technologies such as angioplasty and bone marrow transplants are now commonplace in the USA, many of the health status indicators lag behind those of other industrialized countries (Central Intelligence Agency, 2008). The overall U.S. infant mortality rate is higher than most similarly developed countries because significant areas of the United States lack access to good preventive services. Although highly trained and skilled physicians and nurses work in neonatal nurseries to save the lives of premature babies, prenatal and other preventive care is not available to many pregnant women, resulting in high rates of preterm labor, which ensure fully occupied neonatal nurseries. Dialysis programs are available for people with diabetes who experience kidney failure, but many afflicted with diabetes are unaware of their disease or unable to manage it through diet and exercise. While sophisticated regimens of antiretroviral drug treatment are available for those with HIV infection, many others with HIV/AIDS are undiagnosed and spread the infection through unprotected sex or sharing needles. Twenty-first-century medical technology that is largely confined to health care settings cannot optimize health or prevent disease. This is the role of community-based health promotion.

Focusing health and disease prevention at the community level can be successful only if the community is involved. The World Health Organization recognized the importance of community participation in its definitions of health and health promotion. For example, the definition of primary health care in the **Alma Ata Declaration** reads: "Primary health care is essential health care based on practical, scientifically sound and acceptable methods and technology made universally accessible to individuals and families in the community through their full participation and at a cost that the community can afford to maintain at every stage of their development in the spirit of self-reliance and self-determination" (Mahler, 1981, p. 7).

This understanding of the limitations of the health care system to maintain a healthy population and the contributions to health of the psychosocial and physical environment in which we live has resulted in a shift to a broader community focus (McLeroy, Bibeau, Steckler, & Glanz, 1988). Interventions in community settings differ from individual clinical interventions in their focus on the health of a target population or community. In the targeting of communities for health interventions, community can be considered in one of the two following ways:

- Community as setting, which uses any of the above definitions of community and focuses on changing individual behaviors as a way to lower a population's risk of disease. In this type of intervention, population change is considered as the aggregate of individual, interpersonal, or institutional change.

- Community as target, in which the goal is changing policy or community institutions, such as the development of walking trails, the availability of smoke-free facilities, or the overall rate of a disease.

Whatever the focus, the goal of almost all community interventions is to have an impact on morbidity and mortality factors that occur outside of health care settings. These interventions can be contrasted with clinical interventions, which are individually focused and usually involve diagnosis with physical exam and laboratory tests. This is usually followed by treatment with drugs or procedures, with a goal to prevent an existing harmful condition from becoming worse.

Examples of Community-Based Interventions by Levels of Prevention

Since community interventions involve a vast array of topics, one way of organizing them is by **levels of prevention**. Interventions that focus on **primary prevention** have a goal of avoiding or preventing a disease or condition before it begins. **Secondary prevention** efforts focus on screening and the early diagnosis of a disease or condition. **Tertiary prevention** interventions aim to prevent disease progression after a risk factor or disease has been identified. Table 1.1 provides some initial examples to assist students in identifying a topic area and type of intervention for implementation.

Developing walking can be considered an intervention at both the primary and the tertiary prevention levels because they can be important components in preventing obesity and cardiac disease. They can also be used by people who already have these conditions to help in preventing additional weight gain or further deterioration of cardiac functioning. A school system intervention that seeks to remove soda vending machines from schools is likewise both primary and tertiary in its focus on initially preventing childhood obesity, an important risk factor for the future development of

TABLE 1.1 **Examples of community-based health interventions by levels of prevention**

Intervention	Primary Prevention	Secondary Prevention	Tertiary Prevention
Walking trails	X		X
Removing soda vending machines from schools	X		X
Support groups for breast cancer survivors			X
Back to Sleep campaign	X		
Needle exchange intervention	X		
Know your HIV status intervention	X	X	
Mammogram access		X	
Great American Smoke-Out			X
Buckle-up seat belt publicity campaign	X		

Type 2 diabetes (James, Thomas, Cavan, & Kerr, 2004). Support groups for women with breast cancer have been shown to be effective in decreasing stress and improving coping and overall mental health (Winzelberg et al., 2003). Because the support groups help women to be proactive about potential future complications of the disease process, they are tertiary prevention. The Back to Sleep campaign, jointly sponsored by the National Institutes of Health and the American Academy of Pediatrics, is a social marketing campaign that recommends that infants be placed on their backs to sleep to reduce the incidence of sudden infant death syndrome (SIDS) (Havens & Zink, 1994). This successful primary prevention campaign is credited with reducing the incidence of SIDS 50 percent since its inception in the mid-1990s (National Institute of Child Health and Human Development, 2008).

Needle exchange interventions are a primary preventive measure that can prevent the spread of HIV infection among injecting drug users (Des Jarlais et al., 1996).

Campaigns to increase HIV tests and learn about one's HIV status are considered secondary prevention because of their goals of early detection of HIV infection. They are also a form of primary prevention because of their focus on decreasing the risk of HIV transmission to unknowing sexual partners (Varghese, Maher, Peterman, Branson, & Steketee, 2002). Interventions to increase access to mammograms are secondary prevention because mammograms are an important source of screening for breast cancer (Humphrey, Helfand, Chan, & Woolf, 2002). Women who have their healthy breasts removed because they carry the bracia (SP) gene that puts them at much higher risk of developing breast cancer are practicing primary prevention.

Now that there is a vaccine to prevent the spread of the human papillomavirus, there is a method for the primary prevention of cervical cancer. A campaign to get young women vaccinated is a primary prevention method. Secondary prevention would be a campaign to encourage women to get Pap smears. A tertiary preventive measure is a colposcopy for women who have some abnormal cells (Franco, Duarte-Franco, & Ferenczy, 2001). A buckle-up publicity campaign can be designed to increase seat belt use among the community as a whole, or it can be focused on a target population such as Hispanics or adolescents. Either way, such a campaign is a form of primary prevention against unintentional injuries from motor vehicle accidents (Evans, 1990).

Each of these examples has a citation—that is, each has been shown to be effective in achieving its goals. These interventions are examples of evidence-based practice, in which public health practitioners actually go to the literature and learn if an intervention has been shown to be effective. Such a citation does not guarantee positive results in a given community or population, but the chances of success are much higher than simply making up an intervention de novo or relying on anecdotal experience.

SUMMARY

Public health interventions have a community focus, rather than an individual focus. One of the tasks of public health practitioners is to understand both the composition of the community in which they are trying to make an impact and the level of prevention at which they want to intervene. In the following chapters, readers will be exposed to all the steps necessary to develop a community-based intervention.

KEY TERMS

Alma Ata Declaration

Community

Community-based health interventions

Demographic variables

Ecological theory

Levels of prevention

Primary prevention

Secondary prevention

Target community

Tertiary prevention

ACTIVITY

As discussed in this chapter, communities are not defined solely by geographic boundaries.

1. Identify two examples of nongeographic communities in which you are involved. Describe the commonalities that tie the communities together—such as interests, behaviors, or characteristics.

DISCUSSION QUESTIONS

1. In the United States, the shift of emphasis from infectious to chronic disease has frequently been cited as one of the main reasons for the growing interest in community health interventions. Are chronic diseases better suited to community-based health interventions than other illnesses?

2. Many of the interventions for infectious diseases use strategies involving community networks and organizing. Are these types of community intervention particularly well suited to infectious diseases? What factors influence your response (economics, target population, geography, or others)?

3. How would you identify and define a community in which to conduct an intervention for teen pregnancy? Breastfeeding? Early child development? How would the approach differ between these communities? What are the potential problems that might emerge, depending on the different definitions of the community?

CHAPTER

2

A BRIEF HISTORY OF COMMUNITY-BASED HEALTH INTERVENTIONS

DIANA SILVER

LEARNING OBJECTIVES

- Recognize the aims and objectives of some of the pioneer community-based health interventions
- Relate how the problems in evaluating the impact of large-scale interventions may extend to small-scale interventions
- Understand important issues that can arise in implementing current community-based health interventions

OVERVIEW

This chapter will review the experience of community-based health interventions planned and implemented in the last forty years. It examines the principles and assumptions that underlay early community-based health interventions and discusses some of the problems encountered when measuring their impact.

COMMUNITY-BASED HEALTH INTERVENTIONS: AN INSTRUMENT FOR CHANGE

Community-based health intervention is a relatively recent idea dating to the early 1960s. The phrase refers to the set of interventions designed to create changes in community infrastructure and services, norms, attitudes, beliefs, and policies that would result in improved health status for community residents. While the term is relatively new, the approach is not, and indeed it has guided much of the progress in public health since the nineteenth century. When John Snow removed the handle of the pump from a contaminated well in London in 1849, he was engaged in a community-based health intervention. Faced with recurrent cholera epidemics, Snow was less focused on extending medical care to those who were sickened with cholera and more concerned with addressing the source of the problem.

The planning and implementing of community-based interventions that this volume addresses build on some of the experience of community-based health interventions planned and implemented in the last forty years. Community-based health interventions are concerned with health at the community level—that is, they are designed to create improvements in the overall health status of the community. Their success or failure is measured at the community level, in the *average* change in individuals' health status within a community.

The Rationale for Developing Community-Based Interventions

The rationale for such interventions echoes Snow's orientation. By the 1960s, the dramatic improvements in the health status of populations in industrialized nations had begun to level off, and chronic disease posed a greater threat to health and well-being than infectious disease. Much of the gains in the earlier part of the twentieth century had been due to improvements in sanitation, water, access to food and medicine, and important medical and scientific achievements such as the discovery of penicillin or the polio vaccine. At least in Europe, access to national health care had been established for the vast majority of the population. By the end of the 1960s, Medicare and Medicaid in the United States had established programs that would also extend health care to large portions of the population that had not previously had access. Regulations on chemicals, equipment, and workplace hazards demanded largely by trade unions had reduced health threats to workers. Along with environmental improvements, more consistent access to treatment of both minor and complex health problems had extended life expectancy for men and women of all racial groups, and gaps in life expectancy among racial groups had even begun to narrow.

In the last half of the twentieth century, the leading causes of mortality shifted from infectious diseases to chronic illness, and progress in reducing its impact had begun to slow by the mid-1960s, even as greater understanding of the risk factors for chronic diseases had improved. Considerable resources and attention focused on improving care for those suffering from chronic diseases, with sophisticated technology addressing catastrophic medical events such as heart attacks and strokes. Yet addressing the leading causes of death, especially cardiovascular and respiratory diseases, was seen by the medical community as requiring a change in individual lifestyle and behavior that technology could not address. In contrast, public health practitioners and researchers, in partnership with those in the medical community, began to look to intervening at a community level to address such lifestyle factors.

This chapter reviews the principles and assumptions that underlay five early exemplar community-based health interventions: North Karelia, Stanford Three-Community, Stanford Five-City, Pawtucket Heart Health, and Minnesota Heart Health, all of which addressed some aspect of cardiovascular disease. The major findings of these interventions are reviewed, as well as some of the concerns raised about their implementation and evaluation. The chapter concludes with a discussion of some of the key issues that subsequent interventions have focused on and some that remain for further consideration.

Principles and Assumptions of Early Community-Based Health Interventions

The initial community-based health interventions shared some common assumptions and principles that informed their rationale and design, as well as assumptions about the ways such interventions should work. Following are some of the principles and assumptions that guided the individuals who planned, implemented, and evaluated these interventions.

■ *The focus is on changing **risk behaviors,** not providing treatment.* Although these interventions employed an "upstream" approach, seeking to change norms and behaviors before they resulted in morbidity, they also sought to improve the health of those already diagnosed with chronic health conditions related to heart disease and myocardial infarction. And while they employed various strategies to increase screening and referrals for disease, they were not concerned with developing new treatment or increasing access to health care.

■ *A **population-based approach** is required to address health behaviors.* These interventions embraced the idea that risk behaviors were distributed across the population, with some people at higher or lower risk. Because of the size of the population targeted, even small improvements in risk behaviors could provide big payoffs (Rose, 2001).

▪ *"Community" has geographic boundaries.* The early community-based health interventions defined community as a geographic entity or political jurisdiction. While these communities varied in size, membership was defined as residence within the community. The implementation of community-based health interventions led scholars and practitioners to question and broaden this definition of community, pointing to other meanings of the word (see Chapter One).

▪ *Improved* **case finding** *of those at high risk in the population is important.* A goal of community-based health interventions was to extend the reach of the medical community by identifying those at highest risk. These interventions looked for opportunities to screen for risk factors and ensure that those identified as high risk were attached to a health care provider.

▪ *Individuals are embedded in families.* Some of the strategies these interventions employed were focused on families and aimed to change or reinforce changes in risk behavior on the part of those at risk by enlisting family members in making changes within the household.

▪ *Families are embedded in larger communities that share context and culture, which in turn influence behavior.* Interventions must focus on creating social norms related to health behavior. In addition to seeing individuals as embedded in their families, practitioners also looked beyond the family for other influences on risk behavior and health conditions. They viewed aspects of the physical and social environment as reasonable targets for interventions that would facilitate and reinforce behavior change by changing or shaping norms, values, and attitudes of community members.

▪ *It is possible and necessary to work in many settings at once.* Embracing this assessment of the influences on individual health, the designers of the early community-based health interventions were convinced that programs should be situated within the institutions and other structures in communities. Thus, the early community-based health interventions developed programs in schools, churches, community organizations, health care settings, parks, worksites, stores, and other venues.

▪ *Multiple programs and activities may have a synergistic effect.* While each of these interventions involved multiple strategies and projects, the designers of early community-based health interventions were as interested in the cumulative impact of multiple interventions on an individual's or household's risk behaviors as they were in the ways specific efforts contributed to the overall effect. The interventions, in embracing social context as a determinant of behavior, were intent on working in many arenas—churches, media, health care settings, worksites—with the idea that the interaction of the different interventions would spur new activities and add to the impact of each specific one.

▪ *Interventions can be successfully evaluated to capture the processes and impacts of behavior change.* These early interventions were rigorously evaluated, using **quasi-experimental designs** and employing multiple methods of data collection. Evaluators believed that both **process indicators** and **outcome indicators** could be identified and assessed and that evaluations could provide information on how the intervention worked and what its impact was.

These principles informed the direction and implementation of the set of community-based health interventions initiated in the 1970s and 1980s. Lessons learned from the design, implementation, and evaluation of these interventions laid the groundwork for much of our current thinking about the promise and challenges of community-based health interventions.

EARLY COMMUNITY-BASED HEALTH INTERVENTIONS

The **North Karelia Project** responded to community concern about the high mortality rate from cardiovascular heart disease in this largely rural area of Finland. In 1971, the governor and all parliament members of North Karelia, together with the directors of many voluntary and official organizations, petitioned the Finnish government for funding and assistance to reduce the burden of disease and mortality from cardiovascular disease. In 1972, a new Public Health Act was passed to reorganize primary care in Finland, and leaders from the North Karelia area met with government officials and representatives from the World Health Organization to develop a plan of action (Puska et al., 1985).

The North Karelia Project envisioned a complete community mobilization to alter norms and behaviors that contributed to early mortality of middle-aged men from cardiovascular disease. To achieve their goals, the researchers used varied strategies that combined efforts to inform the public, build skills among women and men, and reorganize the delivery of health care services. They mobilized both health and non-health sectors and looked for opinion leaders both in the medical community and outside it to serve as public ambassadors for the program. Following are some of the activities they undertook:

- Use of mass media (television and print) campaigns to increase awareness and provide information

- Community organizing and mobilization to identify and alter norms and provide support for behavior change

- Mobilization of multiple sectors of society, including health and nonhealth sectors

- Aiming a variety of activities at high-risk and low-risk people, such as smoking reduction support groups, cooking classes, and agreements with local businesses

- Encouraging women to make household changes in the purchasing and cooking of food

- Training of influential leaders whose opinions would permeate down through different levels of society

- Changing the delivery of health care services, which included some formal changes in training and the reorganization of guidelines and materials

In terms of activities within the community, the changes included a reorganization of hypertension control through the hypertension clinics, development of a hypertension register, and a greater emphasis on the organization of follow-up services, especially on patients who had already had a myocardial infarction.

The **Stanford Three-Community Study** was initiated in 1972, the same year as the North Karelia Project, and it also tested a communitywide intervention to change health behaviors that put residents at risk for cardiovascular disease. The Stanford Three-Community Study had substantial input and support from the health care community in its planning and design. While the planning for the intervention carefully investigated norms and attitudes about risk behaviors such as diet, exercise, and smoking, it did not envision a large-scale community partnership across sectors to implement it. Instead, it tested two approaches. In one community, a mass media campaign was undertaken to persuade residents to change their behaviors, accompanied by individual and group education for high-risk individuals. The second community received only the mass media campaign, while the third served as the control group and had no new activities related to cardiovascular disease (Farquhar et al., 1977). The intervention lasted two years, and the three communities were surveyed each year. Initially the community that received the more intensive intervention appeared to have lower levels of risk, especially with smoking, but the difference between the intervention communities declined after two years. At the end of three years, a significant reduction in overall cardiovascular risk was found in both communities receiving the intervention as compared to the control community. The results of the Stanford Three-Community Study were favorable enough to generate enthusiasm for creating a longer, more comprehensive intervention: the Stanford Five-City Project.

The **Stanford Five-City Project** was a six-year intervention (1980–1986) and relied on the use of mass media, as its precursor had, but implemented a more sophisticated approach to media. The program segmented the community into multiple target audiences, crafting messages for each. Program planners used multiple communication channels (newspapers, radio, television, mass-distributed education materials, and correspondence courses) and held a variety of events aimed at reaching and engaging the community (Fortmann & Varady, 2000). These included contests, classes, and workshops for dietary change, the distribution of self-help quit kits to smokers, and support groups. Educational materials were developed using **social learning theory** and tailored to different groups within the community. Two cities, Monterey and Salinas, received the intervention; results from these cities were compared to three comparison cities of similar size and demographic makeup in California.

The results from the project were sobering. As compared to rates in the comparison cities, changes were found in some of the risk factors targeted (namely, blood pressure and smoking) in two communities, but these were far more modest than anticipated. No significant changes between the cities receiving the intervention and the comparison cities were found in exercise, diet, or cholesterol levels during the intervention period, and only small differences were found postintervention.

No changes were observed in mortality from cardiovascular disease (CVD) (Fortmann & Varady, 2000).

Why the disappointing results? Those conducting the evaluation of the project identified several problems with the project and raised questions about the design of such community-based health interventions (Fortmann et al., 1995). They noted that expecting changes in mortality from CVD was unrealistic for a six-year intervention and that change in behavior would be unlikely to be reflected in mortality data for several years postintervention. They also noted that the introduction of new therapies for those with high blood pressure changed the way patients at risk were diagnosed and treated, resulting in better outcomes for these individuals in both the cities receiving the intervention and the comparison cities. Such changes, known as **secular trends**, may have "swamped" whatever effect the intervention had in helping people modify their behaviors.

The **Minnesota Heart Health Project** began in 1980 and ran for six years. The goal of the intervention was to lower the incidence of heart disease and stroke and, like the Stanford study, the focus was on both men and women. Three communities were compared with the target community. Intervention activities were similar to those in North Karelia and included mass media, screening, outreach to health professionals, workshops, and classes. The results showed modest changes in self-reports of behavior modification and modest but positive changes in blood pressure and cholesterol levels. There were no significant morbidity or mortality findings, but there were modest declines for stroke and heart disease in both the target and comparison communities. As in the Stanford study, the effect of secular trends is hypothesized to have masked the impact of the intervention.

The **Pawtucket Heart Health Project**, which ran from 1983 to 1991, focused on reducing stroke and cardiovascular disease rates. The community was mobilized through programs based at worksites, churches, nonprofit agencies, and social service programs. Following are some of the activities of this project:

- Grocery store shelf labeling of low-fat foods

- Installation of a multiple station exercise course in public recreation areas

- Nutrition programs at local library

- Heart health curricula from first grade through high school

- Highlighting of healthy heart foods in restaurant

The community mobilization was coordinated and directed by a hospital and emphasized counseling using social learning theory and referral to medical services. Those at risk were targeted with special activities, as was the general community. There was no media involvement.

The results of the Pawtucket study were

- Increased knowledge of importance of exercise, but no change in reported exercise

- Changes in systolic or diastolic blood pressure in the right direction, but not statistically significant

- Changes in cigarette smoking in the right direction, but also not statistically significant

- Changes in knowledge, but not statistically significant—changes came earlier in English-speaking households, but by 1993 the non-English-speaking households had caught up

- No change in mortality

ASSESSING THE EVIDENCE FROM EARLY COMMUNITY-BASED HEALTH INTERVENTIONS

The evidence across these early interventions was both intriguing and disappointing. Many reviewers have noted that these interventions were complicated and involved coordinating and planning diverse activities (Thompson, Coronado, Snipes, & Puschel, 2003). Other factors that are now seen as having an impact on the results included the long time frame between intervention and health outcomes, the limits of health education in altering behavior, the inadequacy of current health behavior theory for large-scale social interventions, and the difficulties of sustaining changes when they are made (Fortmann et al., 1995). The evaluations of these community-based health interventions all shared four problems in assessing their outcomes.

1. *The effect of secular trends.* Evaluators for these interventions used quasi-experimental designs, choosing other communities as points of comparison. The time frames for these interventions were generally five or more years. In all cases, evaluators noted that their evidence of change was often swamped by the secular trends and medical innovations that contributed to changes in mortality and decreased the relative risk for CVD and coronary heart disease across the nation.

2. *The difficulty of measuring the "dose" of the intervention.* In attempting to understand the impact of these interventions, evaluators struggled to understand the degree to which activities undertaken reached the population at large. Unanswered questions include the following:

- Does there need to be evidence that the intervention has reached the population directly, as in the Stanford Three community?

- Can participation rates be calculated in a meaningful way?

- Are all activities equal in importance, or should some count more in measuring the dose?

- Should environmental interventions that seek to change the context for individuals be measured in this way?

3. *How long should changes in behavior be sustained to declare the intervention a success?* While the North Karelia Project demonstrated changes in mortality sustained over a twenty-year period, evidence of the durability of many of these interventions was more mixed. For example, the Pawtucket Heart Health Project, which demonstrated modest changes in risk behavior at the peak of the intervention, lost those changes three years postintervention. Evaluators and program planners have struggled to define what should be considered impacts in light of such realities (Green, Wilson, & Lovato, 1986; Merzel & D'Afflitti, 2003).

4. *What is a reasonable effect size to expect?* Given the relatively low level of intensity of community-based health interventions, some observers caution that the effect size of 20 to 30 percent change expected in medical interventions or clinical trials is too large (for example, Fishbein, 1996). Yet with little clarity about what to expect, determining the success or failure of these interventions has been subject to debate. Evaluation researchers have sought to weigh the relative costs of these interventions against treating morbidity, while others have suggested other metrics by which to judge such interventions (Mittelmark, Hunt, Heath, & Schmid, 1993). Without guidance about a reasonable effect size, it is challenging to design evaluations that will ensure sufficient statistical power to find effects.

While these problems are not the only ones that make it difficult to fully assess the evidence from these interventions, they present challenges that subsequent community interventions have begun to address. The problems are by no means solved, but these evaluations of early community-based health interventions have raised important methodological questions that the field continues to address.

THE EVOLUTION OF COMMUNITY-BASED HEALTH INTERVENTIONS

Despite the mixed success of these early community-based health interventions, the public health community has embraced such initiatives as a promising approach to addressing health problems. Over the decades that followed these interventions, program planners and researchers have focused their attention on three areas: (1) improving the capacity of communities to plan and implement community-based health interventions; (2) improving existing strategies and activities and developing new ones that can offer substantial payoff; and (3) improving the evaluation of such initiatives with new methods, more sensitive analyses, and new designs that can yield greater insight into the challenges and achievements of community-based health interventions.

Improving Community Capacity to Plan Community-Based Health Interventions

Efforts to have communities consider the role of environmental factors, as well as to design and implement activities to address these factors, led scholars and public health leaders to develop materials to aid communities in their efforts. The Centers for Disease Control and Prevention's **Planned Approach to Community Health (PATCH)** program helped community leaders in assessing morbidity and mortality data; investigating community perceptions; identifying community norms, attitudes, and values; and finding appropriate targets for intervention in the community (Goodman, Steckler, Hoover, & Schwartz, 1993). Though not currently available, the program came in an easy-to-use kit format and was disseminated to communities across seventeen states (United States Department of Health and Human Services, n.d.). The use and implementation of the PATCH approach were assessed in a variety of communities, and evaluators noted the importance of involving a variety of sectors in the community activities and of using both professional and local expertise in developing intervention plans.

Since PATCH, community mobilization and involvement in planning public health activities have become common. Numerous federal programs have integrated such approaches into their efforts (for instance, Healthy Start, CSAP, and REACH). Attention to identifying **key stakeholders** is often a prerequisite for either public or philanthropic funding for such efforts.

More recently, the mix of new and simpler software that can analyze quantitative data about communities has aided the efforts to plan community interventions. Increasingly, data related to health and well-being can be found online, easily downloaded, and manipulated to gain insight into community health problems. The Urban Institute's National Neighborhood Indicators Project (Howell, Pettit, Ormond, & Kingsley, 2003), the Annie E. Casey Foundation's KIDS Count, and a handful of other national philanthropic efforts have pushed community groups, activists, and service providers in communities to systematically use morbidity and mortality data to plan programs. Software programs that can map administrative data at the neighborhood level have been adopted by community agencies and health departments alike. This "democratization of data" has fueled community planning efforts by focusing them on improving the sophistication of their planning.

At the same time, research across a variety of disciplines reminds us of the importance of norms and attitudes on behaviors—a fundamental principle of the early community-based health intervention. Recent evidence of the effects of neighborhoods on adolescent childbearing (Browning, Leventhal, & Brooks-Gunn, 2004) and the impact of schools' racial mix on cigarette smoking (Ennett et al., 2008) and obesity (Bernell, Mijanovich, & Weitzman, 2009) point to new pathways and mechanisms by which peer culture may influence health behavior.

Improving Existing Strategies and Developing New Ones

The early wave of community-based health interventions made use of a variety of psychological theories of health behavior. However, many of these theories were focused on change at the individual level. Newer efforts have focused on using an **ecological theory** to inform interventions and emphasized working at multiple levels within communities (Kok, Gottlieb, Commers, & Smerecnik, 2008). Such efforts have also drawn on insights from the fields of economics, public policy, marketing and communication, political science, and sociology to develop new approaches to changing the behavior of populations. Others have suggested that the principles to guide community-based health interventions should be extracted from evidence of what works (Freudenberg et al., 1994), rather than continuing to implement interventions guided by individual-level theories.

While the early community interventions focused on the links between education, skill building, and behavior change, more recent interventions have sought to change policies and protocols to alter behavior change. Greater attention to regulation and taxation stimulated new approaches to decreasing smoking and car fatalities and making dietary improvements. From providing clean needles to injection drug users to giving low-income families infant car seats, public health policy makers, community leaders, and scholars have examined the impact of providing equipment to aid people to protect themselves against health threats. The public health community has also experimented with changes to policies and protocols in community institutions to address specific health problems, for example, changing the ways in which college administrations view alcohol use on campus or increasing access to sexual education in schools. Advocates for these approaches note that they provide greater opportunity to help communities sustain changes, giving these interventions greater durability than those that relied solely on teaching skills and providing information.

Many of the more recent community-based health interventions have also paid closer attention than previous interventions to the makeup, norms, values, and constraints of particular settings. They have "drilled down" in the community, seeking to better target and tailor interventions to subpopulations, and have focused on the assets and resources in these communities that can be utilized in such interventions. They have paid careful attention to the limits of replicating "best practices," focusing on useful elements of proven strategies. They have focused on the **sustainability** of successful interventions. Thus, they have armed themselves with important political allies, advocating for funding, government intervention, and changes in the private and nonprofit sectors. At the same time, they have called attention to the need to build "community capacity"; that is, to strengthen the capacity of communities to plan and implement new interventions to meet other health threats.

Improving Methods for Evaluating Community-Based Health Interventions

While the evaluations of the early community-based health interventions answered important questions, many questions were left unanswered or answered ambiguously. Evaluators of more recent interventions have sought to develop new approaches to increase the **internal validity** of such designs and improve the utilization of such evaluations.

To peer into the "black box" containing the unanswered questions, community-based health interventions have paid greater attention to specifying the ways in which interventions should unfold and what assumptions are embedded in their plans. Aided by tools for constructing **logic models** (W. K. Kellogg Foundation, 2004) or **change theories**, evaluators have sought to better understand the mechanisms at work in various interventions (see Chapter Five). They have focused on research that gives a fuller picture of the pitfalls of program implementation, noting lessons that go beyond the specific intervention being investigated. In doing so, they have sought to embed the need for evaluation more squarely inside interventions, emphasizing the importance of feeding information back to program planners in a more timely way. To achieve these goals, evaluators have noted the importance of getting program planners involved as stakeholders in the evaluation, participating in identifying the processes they expect to see as their intervention gets underway. The Aspen Institute's *New Approaches to Evaluating Community Initiatives* has been enormously influential in this regard (Connell, Kubisch, Schorr, & Weiss, 1999).

Alongside such efforts, evaluators of community-based health interventions have tried to tackle the measurement of a range of new and familiar constructs that apply to such models. To the degree that community-based health interventions use strategies to address social norms, they have underscored the need to better understand the ways in which such norms operate to impede or facilitate healthy behavior. Evaluators of community-based health interventions have tried to better measure and understand social cohesion. In a somewhat related way, they have pioneered efforts to find ways to measure community capacity reliably and understand its relationship to outcomes of interventions.

In addition to focusing on how to better understand and measure the processes at play in community-based health interventions, evaluators have developed analytic techniques to better understand the ways in which the interventions may achieve their goals. **Multilevel and structural equation modeling** has aided evaluators to address methodological problems that bedeviled earlier interventions. At the same time, some evaluators conducted **utilization research**, focusing on the cost-effectiveness of community-based health interventions (for example, Tosteson et al., 1997), aiding the public health community in assessing how best to spend limited dollars.

Some scholars have focused on securing greater recognition of insights from **qualitative research** into community-based health interventions. Arguing that qualitative research may be more appropriate to adequately capture the social processes that operate within a community, researchers have explored old and new techniques for investigating these processes. As evaluation designs have embraced multiple methods, qualitative researchers have aided in furthering implementation research and interpreting quantitative outcomes. Qualitative researchers have also developed new approaches to giving more timely feedback to those implementing interventions using tools like the **Rapid Assessment Procedure**. These efforts have led evaluators of community-based health interventions away from adherence to particular techniques and toward a broader appreciation for matching methods to the research and evaluation questions asked.

Finally, some public health researchers have sought to build partnerships with communities in directing community assessment, assessing priorities for action, developing interventions, and evaluating them. Advocates of **community-based participatory research (CBPR)** argue that interventions planned by and implemented by community members are more likely to be effective, since they employ community expertise at each stage of the process (Minkler & Wallerstein, 2003). Such approaches have recently been employed in the REACH projects, the most recent set of federally funded community interventions to address diabetes (Collins, 2006).

SUMMARY

This chapter traced the long history of community-based health interventions. It provided a review of the principles and assumptions that underlay five major community-based health interventions that targeted cardiovascular disease: North Karelia, Stanford Three-Community, Stanford Five-City, Pawtucket Heart Health, and Minnesota Heart Health. While the success of these pioneering efforts has been mixed, the lessons learned and recommendations from these initiatives have informed subsequent interventions.

KEY TERMS

Case finding

Change theories

Community-based health intervention

Community-based participatory
   research (CBPR)

Dose

Ecological theory

Internal validity

Key stakeholders

Logic models

Minnesota Heart Health Project

Multilevel and structural equation
   modeling

North Karelia Project

Outcome indicators

Planned Approach to Community Health
   (PATCH)

Pawtucket Heart Health Project

Population-based approach

Process indicators

Qualitative research

Quasi-experimental designs

Rapid Assessment Procedure

Risk behaviors

Secular trends

Social learning theory

Stanford Five-City Project

Stanford Three-Community Study

Sustainability

Utilization research

ACTIVITIES

1. Identify an article on the Multiple Risk Factor Intervention Trial (MRFIT) and on the Hypertension Detection and Follow-up Program (HDFP) and discuss their

similarities and differences in relation to the community-based health interventions described in this chapter.

2. Describe one chronic health condition that appears to have improved over the past twenty years.

3. Considering the information discussed in this chapter, how might future policy be shaped to decrease the incidence of or mortality from a current health problem?

4. Describe one lesson learned from early community-based health interventions that is still applicable and relevant today.

DISCUSSION QUESTIONS

While much work has been done since the pioneering efforts of the early community-based health interventions discussed in this chapter, much remains unknown about these approaches. Discuss the following two key issues:

1. How can the "dose" of an intervention be measured?

2. How do community-based health interventions help the health care community align its resources and priorities with its goals?

CHAPTER

3

ETHICAL ISSUES IN COMMUNITY INTERVENTIONS

LEARNING OBJECTIVES

- Describe the components of a code of ethics
- Enumerate the ways in which community is addressed by the American Public Health Association's Principles of Ethical Public Health Practice
- Become familiar with the role of an institutional review board
- Understand when the use of incentives becomes an ethical concern
- Distinguish between confidentiality and anonymity
- Define vulnerable populations in the context of research participants and specify precautions that must be taken when working with them

OVERVIEW

This chapter covers some of the ethical issues raised in conducting community-based interventions. The material includes guidelines for the **ethical conduct** of research and the use of external academic and nonacademic review boards.

THE INTEGRATION OF ETHICS INTO PUBLIC HEALTH PRACTICE

In the past forty years, the integration of ethical principles into public health research has progressed to the point where ethical considerations now play an important role in every project and study. Prior to World War II, not much thought was given to the ethical issues raised in conducting interventions at the community level. Press reports of the Public Health Service's **Tuskegee Study** on the natural history of syphilis or the Veterans Administration's (VA) hypertension studies brought the lack of concern for the ethical issues raised by community and medical interventions into public scrutiny. In the Tuskegee Study, poor, illiterate African American men with syphilis were recruited into a study on the natural history of syphilis. Researchers continued to follow the men for forty years from 1932 to 1972, even after the discovery of penicillin as an effective treatment for syphilis, and did not inform them about the existence of this drug for their disease (Jones, 1993). In the **VA study,** participants with hypertension were asked to suspend taking the medications that they had been taking. These men were then randomly assigned to one of two groups. One group received the antihypertensive drug treatment and the other a **placebo**. This was done despite the fact that considerable information was available at the time about the benefits of blood pressure reduction through the use of antihypertensive medication. The deaths of several participants resulted in an outcry about the use of placebos in medication trials and resulted in increased scrutiny for all research (Freis, 1967). Reviews of these projects concluded that participants were put at risk of strokes and that more effective controls must be exerted. The legacy of this inglorious history is that it is no longer possible to design, implement, or evaluate a community-based intervention without considering and dealing with the ethical issues raised.

The Development of Professional Codes of Ethics

A **code of ethics** serves as a guide to the everyday professional conduct of practitioners in any specific field. The code of ethics for public health clarifies the distinctive elements inherent in working in community settings and provides a standard to which professionals can be held accountable. A code of ethics is not necessarily comprehensive or static, because new ethical issues arise with changes in the law or technological advances, and thus these codes should not be used as absolute arbiters of ethical disputes. They do provide principles, however, that can be considered in the resolution of such disputes.

Most professional organizations have developed a code of ethics for their membership. The American Public Health Association has developed one that is intended for public health professionals and agencies that work to improve public health and conduct research about the health of the community. The code, or Principles of Ethical Public Health Practice, is based on assumptions held by practitioners in the field. The code includes the following twelve principles:

APHA's Principles of Ethical Public Health Practice

1. Public health should address principally the fundamental causes of disease and requirements for health, aiming to prevent adverse health outcomes.

2. Public health should achieve community health in a way that respects the rights of individuals in the community.

3. Public health policies, programs, and priorities should be developed and evaluated through processes that ensure an opportunity for input from community members.

4. Public health should advocate and work for the empowerment of disenfranchised community members, aiming to ensure that the basic resources and conditions necessary for health are accessible to all.

5. Public health should seek the information needed to implement effective policies and programs that protect and promote health.

6. Public health institutions should provide communities with the information they have that is needed for decisions on policies or programs and should obtain the community's consent for their implementation.

7. Public health institutions should act in a timely manner on the information they have within the resources and the mandate given to them by the public.

8. Public health programs and policies should incorporate a variety of approaches that anticipate and respect diverse values, beliefs, and cultures in the community.

9. Public health programs and policies should be implemented in a manner that most enhances the physical and social environment.

10. Public health institutions should protect the confidentiality of information that can bring harm to an individual or community if made public. Exceptions must be justified on the basis of the high likelihood of significant harm to the individual or others.

11. Public health institutions should ensure the professional competence of their employees.

12. Public health institutions and their employees should engage in collaborations and affiliations in ways that build the public's trust and the institution's effectiveness [Public Health Leadership Society, 2002, p. 4].

Common Attributes of Ethical Codes

The codes of all professional organizations share some common attributes. For example, they all cover respect for individual rights and the protection of confidentiality of participants. Most call for a respect of the diversity of populations. The public health code can be distinguished by its call for universal access to care and for community input into the decision-making process. The primary reason for instituting a code of ethics for community health researchers is that the relationship between researchers and participants is inherently unequal. The practitioner is always an adult and is generally well educated, with a professional degree or some degree of professional status. In addition, by virtue of initiating the community health project, the researcher has an understanding of the overall research process. Participants are more likely to lack a graduate degree, live with the day-to-day reality of a health problem, and have only a minimal understanding of the project into which they are being recruited. A relationship between the researcher and participant can rarely be on an equal footing and brings with it the tension embedded in inequality. Since the balance of power is in favor of the researcher, it is important to consider the potential for the exploitation of individuals, groups, and communities in all facets of the project and establish structures to avoid this potential.

The **ecological level** of the intervention is important in determining many of the ethical issues that can arise. An intervention to address the problem of adolescent drug abuse at the **group level** involves assuring the **informed consent** confidentiality, and safety of participants. Members involved in a school-based focus group examining strategies for a prevention project need to be assured as far as possible that any stories that they relate in the group will not be shared with school officials or parents. Addressing the same issue at the **organizational or community level** necessitates the development of a collaborative relationship, rather than one that feels unequal, as well as assuring that no harmful effects are felt by those participating in the interventions. For example, a drug prevention intervention at a school playground where illicit drugs are bought and sold could result in physical harm to students or staff. Confidentiality might also be an issue if a school or larger community feared that its reputation would suffer were it to be publicly identified as requiring such an intervention. This is not to say that such an intervention should never be undertaken. Rather, the researcher must consider and integrate into the intervention practices that minimize the potential for violence. Finally, in implementing an adolescent drug abuse prevention intervention across schools at the **policy level**, care must be taken to ensure that schools that have the intervention are not somehow stigmatized.

INSTITUTIONAL REVIEW BOARDS

Institutional review boards (IRBs) arose from the concern for individuals enrolled as subjects in research studies and are committees formed at institutions where research is being conducted such as universities, medical facilities, and community organizations. These committees are charged with protecting the rights of the participants who are involved in any research studies. They do this by reviewing research protocols before they are fielded. Since 1974, researchers conducting any federally funded medical or biomedical study require approval from an IRB to proceed (Wood, Grady, & Emanuel, 2002). As a result of this federal mandate, all research—not just federally funded projects—conducted at universities and medical research facilities requires such approval.

The Responsibility of an IRB to Research Participants

IRBs are made up of a group of scientific and nonscientific members who provide researchers with an independent assessment of the ethical issues of a research study. An IRB is responsible for determining and assuring the following:

1. The rights and welfare of participants are adequately protected and they have given their consent to participate after understanding the risks and potential benefits of the intervention

2. The intervention does not place the participants at unreasonable physical or emotional risk

3. The necessity and importance of the intervention outweighs any risks to participants

4. The researcher is qualified to conduct an intervention involving human subjects (Wood, Grady, & Emanuel, 2002)

The Responsibility of Researchers to an IRB

An important component of the IRB process is the necessity for all staff members who will be involved with the design and implementation of the study, data collection, and data analysis to receive training in the **protection of human subjects**. This training involves education about the history of ethical considerations in research and the types of studies that receive exempt status (meaning that there is no possible harm to research subjects), expedited status (meaning that the research involves only minimal risk to the participants), or full review. The training also emphasizes the necessity for maintaining confidentiality. IRB training is available through a university or medical center's IRB office, the National Institutes of Health's Office of Extramural Research (http://phrp.nihtraining.com/users/login.php), or the Collaborative Institutional Training Initiative (www.citiprogram.org/default.asp?language=english).

An IRB will review all aspects of the proposed research, including the methodology, recruitment procedures, consent forms, and survey instruments, usually using a predetermined format. IRB members may have questions about the project and often can offer suggestions for revision that would increase the strength of an intervention and make it more acceptable to the community. Only after all the IRB's concerns have been addressed will the researcher receive permission to begin research activities.

VULNERABLE POPULATIONS

Vulnerable populations in research are those that may not be able to make informed and free decisions about their participation and so are in need of special protections.

These populations include prisoners, developmentally disabled people, pregnant women, and children. Precautions are necessary because there is a history of prisoners and other institutionalized individuals being pressured or incentivized to participate in studies. Currently, if these individuals are to be included in a research study, care must be taken to ensure that the recruitment process is free of any coercion and that no special privileges (such as early discharge or time off of a prison sentence) result from participation (Gostin, 2007).

Research with children must include both formal parental consent and either assent or consent of the children, depending on their age. Younger children who cannot read or write can provide assent by direct questioning or by asking them to point to a graphic that would indicate yes (such as a smiling face) or no (a frowning face). Older children can sign formal consent forms, if indicated by the study material.

While the developmentally disabled have diminished decision-making capacity and a susceptibility to coercion, it is highly desirable for them to participate in research projects directed at their needs. Since the category of developmental disability encompasses a broad range of conditions and subsequent ability to provide consent, the use of both a substitute decision maker along with the individual with the disability can provide some safeguard against coercion (Weisstub & Arboleda-Florez, 1997).

PERMISSION AND CONSENT

To implement an intervention in a community setting such as a church, an emergency room, or a nonprofit agency such as the local chapter of the American Cancer Society, permission to work on a project should be obtained from appropriate organizational representatives. Such permission involves meeting with members of these groups, introducing the research team, and explaining the specifics of the project to be implemented including its goals, risks, and benefits. The community can also be informed about a planned intervention through the media such as local newspapers, radio stations, or newsletters or through groups such as parent-teacher or church organizations. This advance publicity can help to prevent the spread of misinformation. For example, a misunderstanding occurred when a consent form about an interactive HIV/AIDS prevention intervention in secondary schools in Cape Town, South Africa, that involved only an interactive HIV/AIDS drama was misunderstood by some parents as an HIV testing intervention (Mathews et al., 2002). Time and resources must be allocated in community-based research to try several methods of informing the community about the research process. The process of providing information should be bidirectional, and the research team must be prepared to integrate feedback into the final procedures of the research project.

The Consent Form

Potential participants who will be directly involved in any research intervention must understand the risks and benefits of taking part in the project. Their understanding is formalized by the signing of a **consent form** developed by the researcher, generally using a format suggested by their IRB. Consent forms that get all the critical points across to participants in understandable language are not easy to draft, especially if participants are of diverse ethnicity and educational levels. In communities in which English is not the primary language, consent forms must be translated into languages that can be read easily by all potential participants in these communities.

Consent forms must be carefully stored after they have been signed, generally in a locked office or file cabinet. These forms provide a record for the researcher that the participants fully understood the specifics of their involvement in a project and serve to legally protect the researchers and their organization if a participant argues at a later time that she or he did not understand the risks of participation. (A sample consent form for use with respondents appear in the box below.)

Sample Consent Form for Parents or Guardians

You have been invited to take part in a research study about _____. This study will be conducted by *[name of practitioner]*, Department of _____.

If you agree to be in this study, you will be asked to do the following:

1. Complete a questionnaire about your background.
2. Participate in a focus group discussion.

Your interviews will be audiotaped. You may review these tapes and request that all or any portion of the tapes that includes your participation be destroyed.

Participation in this study will take ten minutes to complete the questionnaire and ninety minutes for the focus group discussion.

You will be given a voucher for groceries in appreciation for your participation in this research.

There are no known risks associated with your participation in this research beyond those of everyday life. Although you will receive no direct benefits, this research may help the investigator understand the health needs of_____.

Confidentiality of your research records will be strictly maintained by assigning code numbers to each participant, so that data are never directly linked to individual identity and by keeping all completed forms and tapes in a locked cabinet accessible only to the investigators.

Your responses will be kept confidential with the following exception: the researcher is required by law to report to the appropriate authorities any suspicion of harm to yourself, to children, or to others.

Your responses will be kept confidential by the researcher, but the researcher cannot guarantee that others participating in the focus group will do the same.

(Continued)

(Continued)

   Participation in this study is voluntary. You may refuse to participate or withdraw at any time without penalty. For interviews, questionnaires, or surveys, you have the right to skip or not answer any questions you prefer not to answer.

   If there is anything about the study or your participation that is unclear or that you do not understand, if you have questions or wish to report a research-related problem, you may contact [*name of practitioner*] at [*phone number and address*].

   For questions about your rights as a research participant, you may contact the University Committee on Activities Involving Human Subjects, [*phone number and address*].

   You have received a copy of this consent document to keep.

Agreement to Participate

Subject's signature and date

Consent of a Minor

Parental consent is required if a child—legally defined as an individual under the age of eighteen—is a participant. A number of methods can be attempted to gain consent from parents who may be hard to reach by mail or through the student. These methods can include informational meetings at a community center or the school, where an incentive such as food is provided, or a lottery for those parents who return the form seeking permission for their child's participation, whether or not they agree to participate. It may even be possible to make a home visit to gain parental consent, as long as such a visit is not perceived as coercive.

   There are two types of parental consent: passive and active. In some situations, such as school-based interventions, **passive consent** has been used. This means that if the parents do not sign a form indicating that they object to their child participating in an intervention, it can be assumed that they are willing to let their child be involved. Passive consent has become less acceptable over the past decade because there is no proof that the parents ever read or understood the consent form. Passive consent is no longer permitted in any federally funded research project. Federally funded and government-sponsored research now require the **active consent** of the parents for a child to be able to participate. Active consent means that a consent form is signed by the parents indicating that they agree to their child's involvement. An unfortunate consequence of requiring active consent is that it has become more difficult to get an unbiased sample of the population because it is more than likely that the parents who do sign and return consent forms are more likely to be engaged in their children's activities. The children of parents who do not return consent forms, on the other hand, are often those in greater need of the intervention activities because their parents are less engaged with the child's school.

PROTECTION FOR RESEARCH PARTICIPANTS

Confidentiality means that the researcher knows the names of participants and the community in which the research is being conducted, but will not reveal identifying information to anyone. Participants should not be identifiable through publications or presentations, the media, or any public or private event. All project staff must be trained in the importance of confidentiality; in addition, in situations where participants are able to meet each other, such as in group interventions or focus groups, staff must stress the importance of participants agreeing not to reveal the identities of others or to discuss any of the material from the group. **Anonymity** means identifying information such as names is not collected. If no additional contact with participants will be required and there is no reason to collect names or other identifying information, it is possible to assure participants of anonymity and minimize potential threats of disclosure.

The Use of Incentives

Material items, including cash, food vouchers, phone cards, or film tickets are frequently used as **incentives** to encourage individuals, groups, or communities to participate in an intervention (Hutt, 2003). The decision to use or not to use incentives raises several ethical issues. If the research is being conducted in impoverished communities, the use of incentives which can be manipulative when people are poor, raises the question of whether it is possible to truly gain informed consent if participation is materially rewarded. Incentives can also serve as a deterrent to the future sustainability of an intervention when funding and incentives are no longer available. Conversely, incentives can serve as a way to ensure that a lack of transportation funds or food is not a reason for nonparticipation. The availability of a snack or a meal also contributes to a positive intervention environment for teaching and learning about a health issue. Finally, people's time is limited, and reimbursement for taking up such time is a legitimate way to recruit them into a research project.

In general, the researchers must achieve a balance between an incentive that is substantial enough to attract and retain participants, but not so significant that it fosters resentment in the community between those who are participating in the intervention and those who are not. Incentives should not be so large as to attract participants who are skeptical of the intervention but enroll because of the material gain. For example, to participate in the study a cash incentive greater than the usual hourly wage should probably not be offered to adolescents. Movie or concert tickets may be more appropriate than cash if employment opportunities for teens are scarce. Offering to pay the cost of transportation to and from the intervention and providing a meal or a snack may be enough to draw people into your project.

Protection from Harm

In the implementation of an intervention, an important ethical responsibility is the protection of the target population from harm. For example, in implementing an intervention to increase physical activity among adolescent girls, it would be important to take into account that this population is extremely vulnerable to the development of eating disorders. Awareness of this potential problem will help guide the development of the intervention so that it promotes healthy eating habits. It should also ensure that researchers are alert to early warning signs of problem eating.

Staff must also be protected from harm. This may mean that research staff is not sent into dangerous neighborhoods unaccompanied or without appropriate protection. In situations requiring intensive interviewing about sensitive or disquieting topics, staff should be given time to decompress and discuss the emotional impact of the interview contents.

Respect for Individual Rights

Health interventions at the community level can elicit tension between the perceived need to reduce the risk to the public's health and the rights of the individuals. The policies of the past twenty years to limit smoking in public spaces provide a good example of this tension. Beginning in health institutions and then spreading to worksites, no-smoking policies in some cities now have spread to all public spaces (Tynan, Babb, & MacNeil, 2008). Protection of the public's health from secondary smoke inhalation is now generally viewed as taking precedence over the individual's right to smoke anywhere at any time.

Other situations exist in which **individual rights** trump what many would perceive as an intervention to protect public health. For example, school-based education interventions on the prevention of HIV, pregnancy, or interpersonal violence are generally structured so that if such information runs counter to a parent's personal beliefs, the parent has the right to opt out of their children's participation in the intervention.

ENSURING RESEARCH QUALITY

One way to be certain that the norms and values of a community are respected is to present members of the community with opportunities for input into the design and evaluation of the intervention. A **community advisory board** is a structure that can facilitate a regular two-way exchange of information. Both content and process are important components of such a board. Community members will need education about the methodological requirement of a research study such as randomization or confidentiality, and researchers will need an understanding of why certain topics, questions, or strategies will not work in a particular community. Decisions should be made early in the life of the board about whether a majority decision-making process will be used or one in which community members and researchers reach consensus on issues.

Avoiding Misrepresentation of Findings

A community advisory board can assist in providing valuable feedback about the preliminary findings of an intervention, which can be incorporated into a final report before dissemination to a funding agency or the press. Such a report must be provided in language that is free from scientific jargon. Although some findings will not be appreciated or in some cases accepted by the community representatives, there is almost always something positive that can be reported, even when it is not what was hoped for or expected. Information that could be interpreted in a negative way toward any specific group should be framed so that the underlying causes are clearly understood. For example, in implementing an intervention to increase childhood immunization rates, a finding might be that a higher proportion of certain ethnic groups is reluctant to have their children immunized. One possible explanation that could emerge is that parents of this ethnic group do not properly care for their children. A more likely explanation, however, is that undocumented immigrants are fearful of having their status revealed if they bring their kids to clinics to be immunized. Potential users of services should not be blamed for not using services that are not accessible, affordable, or culturally appropriate. To avoid the misinterpretation of findings, a community researcher can write a press release or an op-ed piece or even hold a press conference to present the findings in an accurate context. This larger context or the fundamental cause, rather than the proximal cause, of a public health problem is critical in the ethical discussion and dissemination of findings.

Community-based interventions will not be successful without the support of the community in general and the participants specifically. For example, an intervention that focuses on adolescent risk behavior may employ young people from the community as peer educators. However, as adults are in control of the intervention, it is their ideas that are most heavily reflected in the research design and implementation. To engage the peer educators more thoroughly in the research, the ideas presented by the peer educators should be incorporated into the intervention and the peer educators should be credited for their contribution. The intervention will receive greater support and will also be more relevant as a result of these ideas.

MAINTAINING THE INTEGRITY OF RESEARCH

At times the interests of the intervention's funder may be at odds with the direction that the intervention is taking. For example, an intervention to decrease teen pregnancy rates by providing teens with knowledge of career options may reveal that it is also necessary to provide them with knowledge about contraception. If the funder is opposed to providing teens with information about birth control, the practitioner is faced with an ethical dilemma, especially if it appears that the funder will withdraw support. In such a situation, the practitioner must make a decision about the best interests of the target community. In this example, it may be possible to have a community agency such as a local clinic or Planned Parenthood provide teaching about contraception to the teens.

Sensitivity to the physical and social environment in which an intervention occurs also raises an ethical issue for community researchers. For example, if an intervention is taking place in senior centers, it is not acceptable to disrupt the routine of all the residents over an extended period of time to carry out an intervention with a few individuals. Nor is it acceptable to take over an area for the intervention that is used by community members as a resource, such as a club or community center. If an intervention involves introducing something new into the environment, such as computers or exercise equipment for the participants to use, then it is ethically preferable to give that equipment to the community when the intervention is concluded.

A community-based health intervention is bound to disrupt some people's lives and introduces a new element into the community. Therefore, it should be methodologically sound, with a scientific rationale for identifying the problem, designing the intervention, and evaluating its impact on the community. The reputations of the practitioners, their organizations, and the community stakeholders who have endorsed the intervention are all dependent on the strength of the maintenance of high ethical standards and careful work.

There are instances when an intervention is not achieving the desired results. For example, the desired change may not be occurring or it may be occurring in an unexpected direction. It might turn out to be impossible to work collaboratively with the community or community agency, or it may turn out that participants are not reflective of the target community. In such a situation, the practitioner must decide whether going on with the project merits the continuing expenditure of funds to support it. The ethical issue here is related to who is going to benefit and who might lose from the project's continuation. If only the practitioner and the staff will benefit, perhaps continuation is not in the best interest of the community. If it is possible to use the funds in a different way to achieve the desired goal, such reallocation may be indicated. Involving community members and using a decision-making process that is as transparent and open as possible can help minimize any bad feelings that might result from the changes.

SUMMARY

A variety of ethical considerations must be kept in mind in the process of planning and implementing any community-based intervention. Receiving formal training, using the resources of an institutional review board, and trying to keep the perspective of the community in mind will help you resolve these considerations in an equitable manner.

KEY TERMS

Active consent

Anonymity

Code of ethics

Community advisory board

Confidentiality

Consent form

Ecological level

Ethical conduct

Group level

Incentives

Individual rights

Informed consent

Institutional review boards (IRBs)

Organizational or community level

Parental consent
Passive consent
Placebo
Policy level

Protection of human subjects
Tuskegee study
Vulnerable populations

ACTIVITIES

1. In the vulnerable populations section of this chapter, several populations are listed. Beyond the reasons listed, identify additional reasons why prisoners are considered vulnerable.

2. Describe one research situation in which true anonymity would not be feasible and why. How would confidentiality then be maintained?

3. In small rural towns in the United States, disclosure of HIV status can seriously affect an individual's standing in the town. Imagine you were working for a countywide AIDS organization and you wanted to conduct a study to better understand the needs of newly diagnosed HIV-positive women in one of the small, rural towns within the county. Describe your approach to conducting ethical research, including

    a. Whether or not you would establish an advisory committee

    b. How consent will be managed

    c. Whether you will choose confidentiality or anonymity, and why you make that choice

4. Imagine you are conducting a study of how homeless individuals in San Francisco access medical care. You are planning on conducting one-time thirty-minute interviews. Describe one reasonable incentive and why it might appeal to this population.

DISCUSSION QUESTION

Review the following case study and discuss the ethical issues it presents and how to deal with them.

The goal of the intervention is to determine whether more high-risk teens will come in for voluntary testing and counseling for HIV/AIDS. Teens will be recruited at one of two high schools in town. Notices will be distributed at places where teens hang out after school, inviting them to come to a mobile van at 11:15 A.M. for voluntary counseling and testing the following Monday through Thursday. After signing a consent form that tells them about the test, all teens will be asked to complete a questionnaire about their sexual activity in the past year. Students who complete the questionnaire and agree to be tested will be given a $50.00 gift certificate after being tested.

Those teens testing negative will have a very short consultation and be given their gift certificate and a pamphlet explaining how to remain negative. Those teens testing positive will be asked to remain in the waiting area for an individual consultation with a social worker and a nurse. After the consultation they will be advised to join a support group and see a physician for follow-up.

Parents or caretakers of the infected teens will be contacted and told about their child's test results within twenty-four hours.

CHAPTER

LEVELS AND TYPES OF COMMUNITY-BASED INTERVENTIONS

LEARNING OBJECTIVES

- Distinguish between primary, secondary, and tertiary prevention interventions in community settings
- Become familiar with differences in community-based interventions at four levels of ecological focus
- Explain the difference between clinical and community-based interventions

OVERVIEW

This chapter introduces students to different types of community-based interventions and provides examples at the different **ecological levels**. Each of these interventions is characterized by a specific prevention and ecological focus, which contributes to the wide range of interventions that public health practitioners can implement.

AN ECOLOGICAL FOCUS ON TYPES OF PREVENTION

A variety of activities have been used to improve health in community settings. These range from education sessions offered to support groups for individuals with a shared condition, to coalitions building to change a community condition, to advocacy for policy and legislative change. In Chapter Three you learned about some of the ethical issues that can arise when implementing an intervention. This chapter will consider the ecological levels in which practitioners work.

Using an ecological perspective, community health practitioners can intervene at any of four levels. At the **group level**, interventions work to change knowledge, attitudes, and practices about a health issue among members of a target group, such as women recovering from breast cancer or new immigrants from Africa. At the **organizational level**, interventions use the shared connection between individuals to build changes in health behaviors and environment. Health promotion interventions at day care centers or work sites take place at the organizational level. At the **community level**, interventions work to change environmental or social structures. Any intervention that enhances the health of people throughout a geographic community occurs at this ecological level. Interventions at the **policy level** change laws or policies that will facilitate health, such as no-smoking bans in restaurants or mandatory seat belt laws.

In addition to the ecological level of an intervention, it is also necessary to determine the prevention focus of the health intervention. Primary prevention interventions concentrate on avoiding a problem or condition before it occurs. These interventions generally work with healthy populations, although they may concentrate on groups at high risk for a condition or disease. Immunization campaigns are an excellent example of a primary prevention activity because they prevent the target disease before any symptoms are apparent.

Primary Prevention

Primary prevention interventions can be implemented at any of the four ecological levels. At the group level, parenting and nutrition education for mothers in a WIC program is an example of a program targeting the prevention of child obesity (United States Department of Agriculture, Food and Nutrition Service, 2005). Implementing a school physical activity program in a school to prevent obesity is an example of an organizational-level intervention (Mo-suwan, Pongprapai, Junjana, & Puetpaiboon, 1998). Working with a local school board to ensure regular physical activities at all schools in the district would be a community-level program to prevent obesity. Helping pass a legislative initiative to assure funding for the construction and maintenance of parks and recreational facilities is a policy-level initiative to prevent obesity.

Secondary Prevention

Secondary prevention interventions focus on the early diagnosis and treatment of a condition. Activities generally revolve around the screening of different populations for a specific disease and ensuring that referral systems are in place for treatment. At the ecological level of groups, secondary prevention might target a group that exhibits risky sexual behaviors to encourage individuals to seek HIV counseling and testing in order to detect disease at an early stage. At the organizational level, secondary prevention of chlamydia might involve establishing a program to ensure the routine screening of all adolescents at a juvenile detention center, because as a group they are at higher risk. An annual HIV testing day is an example of secondary prevention at the community level. Finally, secondary prevention at the policy level for the health problem of sexually transmitted infections could focus on ensuring that adequate funds are available for health departments to conduct routine screening and continue to operate clinics for treatment. While many secondary prevention programs address medical problems and involve collaboration with medical or laboratory facilities for testing and referrals, a behavioral-community example might involve screening for dating violence among adolescents and giving advice on how to end a violent relationship or on changing the aggressive behavior.

Tertiary Prevention

Tertiary prevention interventions work to prevent a diagnosed condition or disease from getting worse and cause the ill individual to develop complications. An implicit goal of all tertiary prevention interventions is to improve the quality of life of the target population. Examples of such interventions might be support groups for veterans returning from combat missions in Iraq with posttraumatic stress disorder to prevent further psychiatric complications, prevention of second pregnancies among adolescent mothers, and physical activity programs for women with cardiac disease to prevent further disease progression. In considering tertiary prevention interventions at the ecological level of groups, an educational program for physicians and nurses in a local clinic about strategies to assure annual foot and eye exams for their diabetic patients can work to change the practices of this provider group. At the organizational level, a hospital-sponsored medication adherence program for all patients who are discharged from the hospital's psychiatric unit will decrease rehospitalizations of patients. At the community level, an example of a tertiary prevention intervention would be a communitywide education program to encourage all diabetics to have annual foot and eye exams to prevent specific complications of their diabetes. At the policy level, the passing of a bill that mandates the development of a program would ensure that all diabetics have access to a glucometer to support better disease control.

SELECTING A GOAL FOR THE INTERVENTION

Before you choose the target population and set goals for a community intervention, it is important to determine both the ecological and prevention focus of the intervention. An intervention addressing primary prevention of HIV infection might focus on condom use among gay and bisexual men (group level); a secondary prevention intervention could encourage access to confidential HIV testing (community level); and a tertiary prevention intervention could focus on ensuring condom availability among men and women who have HIV infection (policy level). It is important to note that the levels of prevention are closely related and lack clear boundaries, so do not be overly concerned in figuring out exactly the level of prevention for your intervention. For example, chlamydia screening in adolescents can be considered secondary prevention for this sexually transmitted infection or primary prevention of pelvic inflammatory disease, which results from an untreated chlamydia infection.

Below are examples of interventions targeting two specific health problems: type 2 diabetes and asthma. Table 4.1 provides an array of intervention ideas focused on adults with type 2 diabetes, and Table 4.2 suggests interventions focused on preventing asthma attacks among children. These interventions represent the wide range of community-based interventions that can be implemented at each ecologic and prevention level.

The decision about which levels of prevention and ecology will be the focus of an intervention will depend on several factors. The first of these factors is the needs determined by the community assessment (see Chapter Seven). Although secondary data may point to asthma, the community may consider teen pregnancy more pressing. The second factor is the current political atmosphere. While the results of the community assessment might show that adolescent pregnancy is an important community issue, local community leaders or advisory boards may not wish to directly address adolescent sexual behaviors. A third factor is access to a population. While it would be ideal to implement an intervention through a community's school system, it may be very difficult to gain access to that system. Finally, the level at which you focus also depends on the resources that are available. While it is possible to create more change with a community-level intervention than a group-level one, working at the community level generally requires greater resources. Similarly, while multilevel interventions tend to be more effective, they are also more expensive and require more experience to design and implement. They also require more time to establish the necessary partnerships.

Practitioners with less experience in developing and implementing community-based health interventions should probably start at the group or organizational level. Community interventions are almost impossible to implement alone, so partnering with others as well as with community agencies provides increased resources, ideas, and access. If limited or no funding is available, decisions will have to be made about whether to spend time recruiting volunteers, fundraising, or starting with a project with a narrower focus.

TABLE 4.1   Health problem #1: adults and type 2 diabetes

	Primary Prevention	Secondary Prevention	Tertiary Prevention
Group	Offer work site education sessions that emphasize lifestyle changes, diet, and exercise to individuals at high risk for developing type 2 diabetes	Offer blood glucose screenings at a local supermarket	Deliver diabetes self-management education for people with diabetes
Organizational	Place signs near stairwells and elevators that encourage employees to take stairs instead of elevators while at work	Implement a work site diabetes screening program for employees	To reduce the burden of vision loss, nursing residents provide early detection and treatment of diabetic eye disease
Community	Launch a social marketing campaign to increase public awareness of diabetes	Implement a communitywide screening program for diabetes	Provide medical staff at all community health centers trainings on how to respond to type 2 diabetes complications
Policy	Establish policies that make physical activity facilities in local schools available to residents after hours	Lobby to pass a bill that increases access to affordable vision screening benefits for Medicare beneficiaries	Develop health policies that improve access, availability, and quality of diabetes care

TABLE 4.2   Health problem #2: preventing asthma attacks among children

	Primary Prevention	Secondary Prevention	Tertiary Prevention
Group	Offer asthma education for members of the local boys and girls club	Provide allergy screenings for kids with asthma at boys and girls club	Provide educational sessions for parents of asthmatic children to ensure that their children have an asthma action plan
Organization	Adapt aspects of a school's environment to remove indoor air hazards that trigger asthma attacks such as dust mites, mold, and pests	Provide spirometry screenings in schools to identify students who show signs and symptoms of asthma	Provide training for school employees on the use of standard emergency protocols when responding to students in respiratory distress
Community	Launch an Asthma Walk campaign to bring attention to asthma and raise funds for asthma research	Offer allergy screenings once a year at all city schools	Develop a training to ensure that all health care providers follow national guidelines when responding to a child in an asthma crisis
Policy	Establish school policies and procedures regarding asthma education and management	Create policy to increase health coverage to include all aspects of asthma screening	Implement policy to mandate that funds be provided to better understand environmental hazards that trigger asthma attacks

EXAMPLES OF INTERVENTIONS AT DIFFERENT LEVELS OF PREVENTION

The following sections present more examples from the literature describing interventions, both successful and unsuccessful, that have been implemented at each of the prevention and ecological levels.

Primary Prevention: Group Level

A Michigan WIC program of 564 women was randomly divided into four groups for the purpose of comparison. One group received a voucher for fresh fruits and vegetables along with education about their importance and use. A second group received only the educational component, a third received only the vouchers, and the fourth received no aspect of the intervention. Education did improve the attitude of the group toward eating fruits and vegetables, although there was little change in their consumption habits. Those who got vouchers to buy fruits and vegetables did increase their consumption, but their attitudes about eating fruits and vegetables did not become more positive. The strongest effect in a change of both attitude and consumption pattern was in the group that received both education about the benefits of fruits and vegetables and the wherewithal to buy them. Anderson and colleagues (2001) conclude that low-income families need both education and financial resources to change their eating habits to regularly consume more fresh fruits and vegetables.

Primary Prevention: Organizational Level

A case study suggests that as obesity becomes more prevalent in the United States, increasing employers' adoption of work site wellness programs could improve employee healthy behaviors, decrease employee absenteeism, and increase employee productivity (Green, Cheadle, Pellegrini, & Harris, 2007). Green and associates describe how Group Health Cooperative, a nonprofit health care system, adopted a ten-week work site wellness program called Active for Life (AFL) to increase physical activity levels among its employees. AFL is an evidence-based program developed by the American Cancer Society that includes goal-setting exercises, self-monitoring practices, economic incentives, and team competitions. Group Health employers implemented AFL after a three-month planning phase. In total, 1,167 out of 3,624 employees participated in the program. Outcome evaluation revealed that while the program increased physical activity levels, such changes were not sustainable. The authors recommended extending or repeating the program, enhancing social support, and providing larger economic incentives.

Primary Prevention: Community Level

Weatherill, Buxton, and Daly (2004) describe a community-based program to increase pneumococcal and influenza immunization rates in a low-income community. Using a geographic definition of community, the team focused on a ten-square-block area to implement a one-month immunization blitz. A storefront was rented, volunteer nurses and community members were enlisted and trained, and a community kickoff and media campaign was organized and implemented. The evaluation of the program showed that 8,723 people were immunized—79 percent with both vaccines. There was a decrease in emergency room visits for pneumonia cases for the three months following the blitz. The final outcome was not clear, because the data were confounded by changes in how and when influenza presented that year.

Primary Prevention: Policy Level

Following the 1995 results of a clinical trial showing that zidovudine given before and at delivery to pregnant women with HIV infection reduced the rate of perinatal transmission by two-thirds, the U.S. Public Health Service and the American College of Obstetricians and Gynecology recommended routine HIV testing for all pregnant women (Centers for Disease Control and Prevention, 1995). This policy resulted in a decrease in perinatal HIV transmission from 2,000 births in 1992 to fewer than 200 a few years after implementation (Fowler, Lampe, Jamieson, Kourtis, & Rogers, 2007).

Secondary Prevention: Group Level

Kalichman and associates (2001, 2005) describe a theory-based group behavioral skill-building intervention to reduce HIV-transmission risk behaviors among HIV-positive people. Individuals (223 men and 99 women) were randomly assigned to receive either five 120-minute sessions that focused on development of skills found to influence high-risk sexual practices or five 120-minute sessions that focused on providing social support (such as HIV information, disease and treatment management, insurance concerns, and nutrition). The group members receiving the skills-based behavioral intervention were less likely to engage in unprotected sex and more likely to use a condom than group members who had not received the behavioral intervention. The authors conclude that group interventions that include couple support and behavioral skill building can be effective in reducing risky sexual behaviors among people living with HIV.

Secondary Prevention: Organizational Level

McCaw, Berman, Syme, and Hunkeler (2001) describe how a nonprofit managed care facility was able to increase screening for domestic violence, improve awareness of the facility as a resource for domestic violence, and improve member satisfaction with the ways in which the facility addressed domestic violence. The first phase of the project focused on infrastructure development in the form of provider training and community linkages to have services in place *before* efforts to increase referrals were initiated. The second phase of the project provided in-service training to all staff about resources and screening, together with environmental cues such as posters, resource cards, and educational materials in waiting areas. Domestic violence referrals increased 260 percent, from 64 in the period before to 134 in the period after the program. Member surveys pre- and post-program showed statistically significant changes in remembering questions asked about family problems, awareness of information on the part of the organization, and overall satisfaction with the organization's efforts to address domestic violence.

Secondary Prevention: Community Level

A coordinated community-based diabetes screening program was implemented in hospitals, health departments, home health agencies, and work sites across the state of Michigan for a six-month trial period (Tabael et al., 2003). Of the 3,506 individuals screened, 14 percent did not meet the screening guidelines, 91 percent reported having a primary care provider, and 11 percent reported a previous diagnosis of diabetes. While the screening instrument identified 57 percent of those screened as being at high risk of diabetes, only 5 percent had positive blood tests. The authors suggest that inappropriate screening and the high false positive rate of the screening instrument make screening of the general population a poor use of resources.

Secondary Prevention: Policy Level

Breast cancer is the second most prevalent form of cancer occurring in women, and while there is no proven method to prevent breast cancer, early detection can improve treatment outcomes and quality of survivorship (American Cancer Society, 2007). Underserved and uninsured women have had limited access to this diagnostic service due to lack of health insurance or restrictions on health insurance coverage. In 1990, to increase access to screening services for these women, Congress passed the Breast and Cervical Cancer Mortality Prevention Act, which authorized the Centers for Disease Control and Prevention to establish the National Breast and Cervical Cancer Early Detection Program (NBCCEDP). Currently, NBCCEDP funds programs throughout the nation, providing screening services to women at risk. To date, these programs have reached 3.2 million women, providing more than 7.8 million breast and cervical cancer screenings (Centers for Disease Control and Prevention, n.d.).

Tertiary Prevention: Group Level

A group of women with breast cancer were randomly assigned to participate in a twelve-week web-based breast cancer support group called Bosom Buddies, which provided moderator-facilitated discussions on twelve topics related to breast cancer. Support group members were also able to access online testimonials from breast cancer survivors, post their own breast cancer story, and keep a personal online journal. Compared to women who did not participate in the web-based breast cancer program, Bosom Buddies participants demonstrated an improvement in depression measures and a reduction in perceived stress scores (Winzelberg et al., 2003).

Tertiary Prevention: Organizational Level

Multisystemic therapy (MST) is a tertiary-level ecological intervention to prevent recidivism among delinquent youth that has been included in the Center for the Study and Prevention of Violence Blueprint Series of scientifically validated violence prevention programs. The MST program emphasizes changing the social ecology of adolescent offenders and their families and operates in the home, school, and community environments of the involved youth. The program is adopted throughout a school system and provides intensive family-based supports, services, and intervention to prevent out-of-home placements. Intensive supervision, interagency collaboration, and consultation are also key components of the MST model. The systemwide implementation of MST has been shown to be effective in decreasing delinquency and truancy. Implementation, however, requires school systems to invest substantial amounts of time and effort (Schoenwald, Brown, & Henggeler, 2000).

Tertiary Prevention: Community Level

Smoking-specific activities were implemented in three pairs of matched communities as part of the Minnesota Heart Health Program (Lando et al., 1995). Activities in the intervention communities included adult education programs for cessation, contests, classes, self-help materials, telephone support, and home correspondence programs. The results showed no effect on men and only minimally positive effects on women. The authors cite two reasons for the disappointing results: a larger-than-expected secular trend occurring in society as a whole and many activities targeted to hard-core smokers, which had minimal effect on the population prevalence.

Tertiary Prevention: Policy Level

To reduce blood-borne disease transmission among injection drug users (IDUs), New York state passed the Expanded Syringe Access Program (ESAP), which authorizes the purchase of nonprescription syringes by IDUs aged eighteen years and older from pharmacies that have voluntarily registered with the New York State Department of Health (Fuller et al., 2007). Because previous studies had identified police harassment, poor needle supplies, limited operating hours, and long travel distances as barriers to syringe access for IDUs, program planners anticipated that the use of pharmacies as a source for safe needles would reduce barriers to using sterile syringes. In addition, participating pharmacies could provide IDUs with education about safer sex practices and serve as a needle disposal site, thus decreasing risk of diseases related to unsafe sex practices as well as needle-stick injuries. Recently, Fuller and colleagues (2007) conducted a study to determine the impact of deregulating pharmacy syringe sales in New York. Evidence from this study indicates that although pharmacies have been approved for syringe dissemination, their participation in ESAP is minimal because of concerns about selling syringes to IDUs (Fuller et al., 2007).

SUMMARY

This chapter has described different prevention and ecological levels for health interventions. Primary, secondary, and tertiary level interventions focus on problem prevention, early detection, and amelioration, respectively. While these intervention levels reflect the different approaches that can be taken to address health issues, ecological levels describe the population focus for health interventions. Citing studies published in peer-reviewed journals, this chapter presented strategies that have used group-level interventions to target aggregates of people who share common characteristics; organization-level interventions, which target groups bound by common interests, work, or goals, such as work sites; community-level interventions, which take place in the context of a neighborhood; and policy-level interventions, which influence the systems affecting neighborhoods and the people who live in them.

KEY TERMS

Community level
Group level
Organizational level
Policy level

Primary prevention
Secondary prevention
Tertiary prevention

ACTIVITIES

1. Select one health problem not discussed in this chapter and identify potential primary, secondary, and tertiary prevention interventions that might be conducted at each of the four levels of ecological focus.

2. Design a primary prevention plan to reduce deaths by firearms among teenagers.

    a. On which ecological level would the intervention focus?

    b. Describe one potential strategy for each ecological level.

3. Describe one recent intervention at the policy level that resulted in change. Identify one popular media source (such as a newspaper or magazine article) and one scholarly article (such as a policy brief or peer review journal article), and write a few bullet points describing the policy.

    a. How and when did this policy shift occur?

    b. Who were the key contributors that enacted the policy change?

    c. Who is the target audience of the policy?

    d. What measures are in place to monitor effectiveness?

DISCUSSION QUESTIONS

1. Imagine you are a program administrator for a city health department. You have recently been charged with developing a program targeting cardiovascular disease and need to decide if you will devote your agency's resources to designing a group-level intervention, a community-level intervention, or an intervention that operates at both the group and community levels of the ecological model. Of

the three choices, which will you select? Explain your answer and the factors that contributed to your decision.

2. A health agency is interested in planning an intervention that addresses adolescents and tobacco use. They want to use primary, secondary, and tertiary interventions at each ecological level. Fill in the following table and note the difficulties you had in providing examples for each cell. Were certain cells more difficult to fill than others? Explain your answer.

Health problem: adolescent smoking

	Primary Prevention	Secondary Prevention	Tertiary Prevention
Group			
Organization			
Community			
Policy			

PART

2

DEVELOPING THE INTERVENTION

5

A FRAMEWORK FOR DESIGNING COMMUNITY-BASED INTERVENTIONS

LEARNING OBJECTIVES

- Understand the purpose of using a theoretical framework for a community intervention

- Define the key constructs of one group-, one organization-, one community-, and one policy-level theory used to guide community-based interventions

- Describe the relationship between theoretical constructs and intervention activities

OVERVIEW

The purpose of this chapter is to expose students to the different types of **theoretical frameworks** that program planners can use to design and implement community interventions.

THEORETICAL GUIDANCE FOR HEALTH INTERVENTIONS

Community health interventions must do more than educate or provide knowledge to a target population about a desirable behavior. Excellent evidence is available to demonstrate that knowledge alone will not change an individual's behavior. For example, how many readers have good knowledge about eating low-fat and low-calorie foods, exercising daily, using sunscreen, and practicing safe sex, yet do not regularly practice these behaviors? Therefore, an intervention must incorporate components or activities in addition to educational activities to change behavior. By providing a construct made up of various components, a **theory** provides guidance as to what program activities could be included to reach your goal.

Theoretical Models

Successful community interventions do not just spring up from the desks of practitioners. Most will use a theoretical model to develop the activities of an intervention to change a targeted health behavior. Most of the theories used in health promotion interventions are from the behavioral sciences and require knowledge of health sciences, epidemiology, and cultural competence to be applied to interventions to address a community health problem. A theoretical model or framework—the terms are used interchangeably here—provides an organized way to think about behavior change and view the set of relationships between a health problem, a target population, program components, and program results. Because the application of a theoretical framework requires practitioners to specify their goals, activities, and outcomes and think through how each of these affects the other, interventions that are based on a theory are more likely to be successful.

Any discussion of theory necessitates an understanding of three particular terms: a **concept**, a **construct**, and a **variable**. A concept is the building block of a theory. Each concept corresponds to a specific construct, and a variable that operationalizes (measures) the construct. For example, one of the main concepts of social cognitive theory is that a person must feel confident that she can implement the desired behavior—that is, exercise self-efficacy about her ability. **Self-efficacy** is, therefore, the theoretical construct that defines the concept. An intervention that aims to increase physical activity can apply a theory in which self-efficacy is a construct to measure participants' sense of confidence in the likelihood of starting to exercise. To **operationalize** the construct, questions will be developed such as, "How sure are you that you will be able to walk for twenty minutes each day?" and "How certain are you that you will attend an aerobic dance class once a week over the next six months?"

Theories provide a mechanism to assess the precursors of behavioral change. While it may be difficult for a one- or two-year (or even shorter) intervention to change the incidence (rate) of dating violence in a high school, use of a theory allows program planners to measure the precursors of dating violence, such as participants' self-rated ability to prevent dating violence. Another example with a similar target population, high school girls, would be an intervention to reduce adolescent pregnancy rates in the target community. While an intervention implemented in one school over a relatively short period of time will not be able to clearly demonstrate such a change, measuring willingness to use condoms or a desire for future life goals are theoretical precursors to changing adolescent pregnancy rates.

The Constructs of Theory

In applying a theory, each of the activities of an intervention should reflect or be developed from one of the constructs or building blocks of the theory. For example, assume that theory X posits that knowledge, skills, and access are key constructs for behavior change. Therefore, an intervention using theory X whose goal is to decrease emergency room visits for asthma among African American children in a targeted elementary school would have intervention activities to reflect this theory. The link between the constructs and the intervention activities might look like those in Table 5.1. Of course, knowledge of health sciences, children's developmental level, and cultural competence should also be integrated into all intervention activities.

TABLE 5.1   **Key constructs and intervention activities**

Key Constructs	Intervention Activities
Knowledge	Book at appropriate literacy level featuring how an African American family works with its children who have asthma
	Laminated colorful instruction sheet with instructions on inhaler use; refrigerator magnet listing the danger signs that indicate necessity of an ER visit
Skills	Interactive teaching sessions with children demonstrating inhaler techniques
Access	Back of laminated instruction sheet has list of local clinics and primary care providers, contact information, and hours

Measurement of Theoretical Constructs

The use of a theory provides an organizing principle for the intervention's implementation and evaluation by forcing the development of a logical relationship between the constructs of the theory, the program's activities, the variables that will be measured in the evaluation, and the hypothesis. Each of the constructs of the theory should be measured as one of the variables in the model. Generally, theoretical constructs are predictor variables, because we hypothesize that they will lead to behavior change. The researcher will also measure the outcome variable—usually the behavior or behavioral precursor that is predicted to occur as a result of the intervention.

In the preceding example, the predictor variables would be

- Knowledge about asthma and inhaler use

- Knowledge about local providers

- Skills in inhaler use

- Access to and use of non-ER providers

The outcome variable would be ER visits at the local hospital for asthma by the target population. The main hypothesis would be *Participation in the XYZ intervention will result in a decrease in ER hospital visits for asthma-related conditions.* Subhypotheses would be *Participation in the XYZ intervention will result in increased knowledge about asthma, increased knowledge about and use of local providers, and improved skill in inhaler use technique.*

EXAMPLES OF THEORIES USED AT THE FOUR ECOLOGICAL LEVELS

Theories are available to direct interventions and change health behaviors in one of the four different levels of the ecological model: group, organization, community, or policy. Group-level theories focus on the social environment and the interactions between individuals. Organization-level theories focus on changing an organization's structures, functions, and practices. Community-level interventions focus on moving groups' shared interests (such as those of African American men), activities (such as those at elementary schools in the district), or geographic areas, generally through the use of communication theories or participatory approaches. Policy-level theories focus on influencing the context and processes that play a role in the development and implementation of policies.

Intervention Theory for Group-Level Change

Social cognitive theory focuses on the fact that people learn by observing the behaviors of others and that such learning occurs on both a cognitive and a social level (McAlister, Perry, & Parcel, 2008). The theory is based on six key concepts that are explained in Table 5.2.

TABLE 5.2   **Six key concepts of social cognitive theory**

Concept	Definition	Examples
Reciprocal determinism	Bidirectional interaction between individual and environment: Actions of individuals influence their environment, and individuals can change environments to have a positive influence on health Environment can either facilitate or block healthy behavior	Individuals lobbying to pass legislation providing federal resources for Pap smear, mammography screening, and treatment services (policy or environment) for low-income, uninsured women, which after a period of time increased the number of women eligible for targeted services (environment having a positive effect on health-seeking behavior) Removing ashtrays from house if trying to stop smoking Avoiding contact with drug-using friends if trying to stop drug use
Behavioral capability	Knowledge and skills to implement a desired action	Low-income, uninsured women are aware of mammography and Pap smear resources Students correctly demonstrate how to put a condom on a penis model Role-playing of responses to common reasons for not wanting to use condoms
Expectations	Probability of a desired outcome from performance of behavior	Understanding that mammography increases the likelihood of early detection and successful treatment of breast cancer Understanding that others have stopped smoking or using drugs

(Continued)

TABLE 5.2   **Six key concepts of social cognitive theory (*Continued*)**

Self-efficacy	Belief in one's ability to perform a particular action	Belief in one's ability to be a user of mammography services
		Feeling confident enough to ask partner to use condoms
Observational learning	Interactive knowledge transmission	Influential others (such as female family members, friends, and co-workers) use mammography services
		Friends have stopped smoking or using drugs
Reinforcement	Use or practice of desired behavior by influential others	Mammography practice of an influential person in the community leads to the early detection of cancer
		Influential sports figure discusses how his stopping drug use increased his performance

Applying social cognitive theory gives researchers the concepts shown in Table 5.2 to develop intervention activities that will meet research goals. (For additional information on social cognitive theory, go to www.tcw.utwente.nl/theorieenoverzicht/Theory%20 clusters/Health%20Communication/Social_cognitive_theory.doc.)

An example of the application of social cognitive theory is the work of Winkleby, Feighery, Altman, Kole, and Tencati (2001), who conducted an empirical study to determine whether direct interventions such as advocacy trainings could influence self-efficacy and affect individuals' motivation to engage in the political process. The researchers used social cognitive theory constructs of perceived self-efficacy to engage in community activities, perceived incentive value, and outcome expectancies. They developed an intervention carried out as a weekend advocacy institute and ninety-minute meetings offered throughout the school year. Participants included 116 adolescent high school students from low-income neighborhoods. Demographic information determined that the sample was predominantly female, with an average age of fifteen, and ethnically diverse (36 percent Asian or Pacific Islander, 22 percent Latino, 7 percent African American, 6 percent white, and 29 percent mixed ethnicity). In order to assess the social cognitive theory constructs of self-efficacy, perceived incentive value, and outcome expectancies associated with participation, the researchers administered a fifty-item pre- and post-test that measured number of activities involved in community advocacy, community advocacy constructs of perceived incentive value, outcome expectancies, perceived self-efficacy, perceived policy control, leadership competence, sense of community, and substance use (tobacco, alcohol, and marijuana). The analysis assessed pre versus post differences for community advocacy activities and constructs.

The investigators found significant differences among both boys and girls for involvement in community advocacy activities; perceived self-efficacy, as well as perceived incentive value, significantly increased for girls; leadership competence increased for boys; and perceived self-efficacy and sense of community approached significance for boys. In addition to the community advocacy projects carried out by the teens, the youths successfully achieved policy-level changes. The researchers concluded that as a result of specific training individuals can be motivated to effectively impact public policy.

Intervention Theory for Organization-Level Change

The **stage theory of organizational change** provides a framework for us to understand how and why organizations initiate, implement, and evaluate new programs. While based on Prochaska and DiClemente's (1983) stages of change theory—a theory that examines individual behavior change—this theory's focus is on the organization, not the individual. The stage theory of organizational change is based on the work of Lewin (1952), who described factors resisting and facilitating change in organizations, and on diffusion theory (Green, Ottoson, Garcia, & Hiatt, 2009), which describes how knowledge is translated into practice. Stage theory hypothesizes that the change process for an organization involves the following seven steps:

- Awareness of unsatisfied demands in the system: some part of the system receives information indicating a problem or potential problem

- Search for possible responses, as elements in the system try to find alternative solutions

- Evaluation of the various alternatives

- Decision to adopt a course of action, which is selected from the options evaluated; operational goals and means are also adopted

- Initiation of action within the system with the formulation of a policy or other directive for implementing the change and the acquisition of resources necessary for implementation

- Implementation of the change; resources are allocated for implementation and the innovation is carried out

- Institutionalization of the change as the innovation becomes part of routine organizational operations (Beyer & Trice, 1978)

In their review of HIV/AIDS system-level interventions, Bauermeister, Tross, and Ehrhardt (2008) found three different types of strategies for organization-level change: technical assistance, infrastructure development, and external partnerships. Interventions that focused on infrastructure development included skill-building activities for providers and staff, organizational restructuring, and improving access to resources. Technical assistance programs focused on skill-building activities for program planning, intervention implementation, community outreach, and service delivery. These studies used both internal and external indicators as outcomes. Interestingly, the technical assistance studies of Kelly et al. (2000, 2004, 2006) found the most effective strategies were those using a variety of teaching modalities together at one site. The infrastructure development studies reported outcomes ranging from changes in available programs, in staff skill levels, in client health behavior, and HIV/STI (sexually transmitted infection) prevalence markers. Interventions that focused on external partnerships included coalition building, community mobilization, and service bundling. The outcomes of these studies were changes in client behaviors and HIV/STI prevalence markers.

Another example of a system-level intervention is the work of Smith, Steckler, McCormick, and McLeroy (1995), who adapted a four-stage model of the theory—awareness, adoption, implementation, and institutionalization—in their work of disseminating curricula about tobacco prevention into school systems. In the awareness phase, they presented information about different curricula at state conferences that were mandatory for school administrators and teachers and followed up with site visits to each district. Several follow-up visits were required for some districts. For adoption, administrators were offered a choice of several tobacco cessation curricula. A champion or supporter was found to be necessary at each of the districts that agreed to implement a curriculum. For implementation, a variety of training sessions were held. Larger school districts and those with health coordinators were able to implement more easily than smaller districts and those without supportive staff. In the institutionalization phase, the researchers learned that it would be difficult to maintain the curricula in their present form. Their analysis of lessons learned included challenges from staff turnover, lack of perceived importance of health education, school pressure to offer a variety of prevention programs, and curriculum not delivered as trained or by teachers without training (Smith et al., 1995). Their experience suggests the need for buy-in by insiders who can provide researchers with the knowledge about the day-to-day workings of an organization or system, which will be critical for the success of any health intervention.

Intervention Theory for Community-Level Change

Social marketing is a communication theory frequently used in health promotion programs. A program based on social marketing involves the "design, implementation, and control of programs seeking to increase the acceptability of a social idea or practice in a target group" (Kotler, 1975). Such programs apply the successful principles of product marketing to health behaviors conceptualized to be in the best interests of a target group or the larger society and include ideas such as acceptance of family planning or a product such as condoms. Social marketing programs involve the use of **five Ps:** *product, price, place, promotion, and positioning.* Strategies such as market segmentation, consumer research and communication, and advertising techniques such as the five Ps are used.

A campaign to increase both community and occupational safety in Alberta, Canada, used a social marketing approach. The campaign was based on an injury monitoring program that was located initially in the local hospital and later with the regional health department. After completion of a community survey on attitudes and behaviors that provided baseline information to be used to assess effectiveness, the following intervention elements were implemented:

- Development of a mascot—a green plush Safetysaurus—who provided a visual identity for the project (positioning)

- Cable television public service announcements (placement)

- School programs (promotion)

- Community safety audits (promotion)

- Community animation in which city government, school boards, the local hospital, fire department, Chamber of Commerce, and library agreed to coordinate educational messages and programs to maximize effectiveness (product, promotion) (Guidiotti, Ford, & Wheeler, 2000)

While a formal assessment of the demonstration project is not available, the preliminary evaluation resulted in Fort McMurray becoming the first North American city to gain entry into the World Health Organization's Safe Community Network.

A second example of social marketing is the paid and unpaid campaign to increase awareness, knowledge, and daily consumption of folic acid among Hispanic women in the United States (Flores, Prue, & Daniel, 2007). The campaign consisted of unpaid Spanish-language public service announcements (placement) about folic acid (product) and a paid Spanish-language media education campaign (promotion) about the value of a healthy baby (positioning) in selected U.S. market cities (place) in 2000 and 2002. The analysis compared the pre- and postcampaign survey results from questions on knowledge of, attitudes about, and use of folic acid among a population of Spanish-speaking Hispanic women contacted through computer-assisted telephone interviews in both intervention and comparison communities. The results of the data analysis showed increases in the three outcome areas of interest with both campaigns; however, significantly greater increases were seen in the paid than the unpaid campaign. (Further information about social marketing theory is available at http://depts. washington.edu/obesity/DocReview/Hendrika/basedoc.html.)

Intervention Theory for Policy-Level Change

The **advocacy coalition framework** provides a model for understanding the processes involved in implementing policy-level social change and is especially applicable to health issues that engender strong public opinions, such as restrictions on the use and sales of tobacco and alcohol (Weible, Sabatier, & McQueen, 2009). Figure 5.1 is a structural diagram of the different constructs of the framework, which includes "policy participants from all levels of government, multiple interest groups, research institutions, and the media" (Weible & Sabatier, 2006, p. 124). Application of the framework requires a period of at least ten years, an understanding of subsystems, the involvement of multiple levels of government, and an understanding that belief systems can change priorities and policies.

The impact of feminist ideas on domestic violence policy in two local municipalities of Canada was examined by Abrar, Lovenduski, and Margetts (2000). These authors document the development of a broad-based coalition of feminists that came together beginning in the 1970s to change legal outcomes and practice for women who were involved in domestic violence situations. The coalition's gender analysis, which understood domestic violence as a function of male domination, was countered by a

FIGURE 5.1 *The advocacy coalition framework*

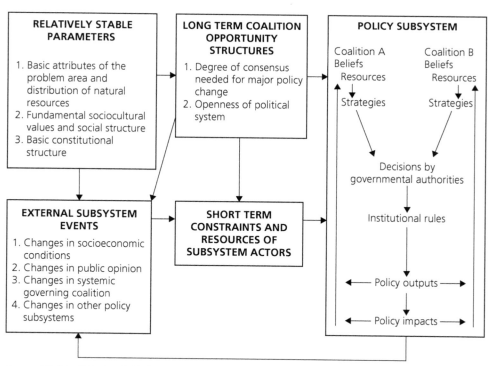

Source: Weible, Sabatier, & McQueen, 2009

traditionalist coalition with a core belief in the sanctity of family life. Activities used to implement change in domestic violence policy, laws, and practices included public and legislative education, research, cultural productions, public demonstrations, intra-agency work groups, and inclusion in academic materials. These activities provide an excellent example of the many levels at which it is necessary to implement interventions to change policy.

SUMMARY

Most theories used in health promotion interventions are from the behavioral sciences. Theories are a set of interrelated concepts, constructs, and variables that explain behavior, suggest ways to achieve behavior change, and provide practitioners with the ability to measure the change process of participants in an intervention. When you use a theory to guide intervention development and evaluation, you must take care to ensure that activities correspond with specific constructs. Different theories are suited to different ecological levels. The theories discussed in this chapter apply to the group, organization, community, and policy levels of the ecological model.

KEY TERMS

Advocacy coalition framework
Behavioral capability
Concept
Construct
Expectations
Five Ps
Observational learning
Operationalize
Reciprocal determinism

Reinforcement
Self-efficacy
Social cognitive theory
Social marketing
Stage theory of organizational change
Theoretical frameworks
Theory
Variable

ACTIVITY

Select one theory from among those discussed here or a theory that is commonly used in health promotion. Conduct an electronic search of the literature to identify a published journal article that documents an intervention in which practitioners used your identified theory to guide their decisions in intervention planning and evaluation. Develop a presentation that

1. Describes how your selected theory's key concepts, constructs, and variables are believed to explain health behavior

2. Provides a description of your identified intervention with attention to the ways in which the practitioners used the theory to guide their intervention development, implementation, and evaluation

3. Briefly discusses the ecological level at which the intervention operates

DISCUSSION QUESTIONS

1. Discuss the role that theory plays in planning, implementing, and evaluating community-based health interventions.

2. Describe how to apply the constructs of social cognitive theory to community-based health interventions.

3. What limits do you see in the theories presented in this chapter? Discuss these limits using a case example of your choice.

CHAPTER

6

COLLECTING AND MANAGING DATA

LEARNING OBJECTIVES

- Explain the difference between primary and secondary data
- Describe the variety of methods used to collect both qualitative and quantitative data
- Recognize the key aspects necessary for successful population sampling
- Become familiar with the basics of compiling a questionnaire
- Understand the steps needed to prepare both quantitative and qualitative data for analysis

OVERVIEW

This chapter discusses the ways data are used to establish needs and determine whether objectives are being met in community interventions. The chapter also covers how to prepare for the collection of both quantitative and qualitative data, the tools needed to collect the data, and ways to prepare the data for analysis.

DATA: A CRUCIAL COMPONENT OF RESEARCH

Data are collections of pieces of information that can be organized in a way to increase knowledge about something of interest. They consist of pieces of information that can be identified from facts collected in a variety of ways including observation, people's responses to questions, or laboratory experiments. Data about the same attribute or event can be combined together to form a **variable** such as social class, which is commonly a combination of an individual's educational level, occupation, and income. A **data set** is a collection of variables related to a specific topic such as adolescent risk behaviors or state health care expenses in a given year. **Data processing** converts the collected information into a usable form such as numbers that are used as a code for pieces of information so that the information can be manipulated into variables and ultimately new knowledge.

Why Collect Data?

Data are necessary to support the rationale for and evaluation of proposed interventions targeting risk factors or health conditions that practitioners view as requiring attention. Data collected from the same source over time can indicate whether an intervention is having the expected results. Not only are data needed to determine whether an intervention is necessary, but data collected through interviews with community leaders will indicate whether the intervention is likely to be supported by the community. After implementation of an intervention, data are needed to determine whether the intervention successfully reached its aims and objectives. Data are used to persuade funders and policy makers to support an intervention. Decisions to grant funding for projects are to a large extent based on the strength and validity of the data indicating need. Data must be valid and carefully collected because they are likely to be quoted in public documents such as newspaper articles and reports about a project.

Types of Data

Primary data contain new information that has not been previously analyzed. **Secondary data** are data that have already been collected by someone else, including **large data sets** available at the web sites of the National Center for Health Statistics, the National Institutes of Health, the Centers for Disease Control and Prevention, or local health departments. These secondary data sets are often available to the public for analysis. These data sets and other previously collected data can offer incidence and prevalence rates on the condition generally and possibly rates in the community in which an intervention is planned.

Data can be collected in the form of both numbers and words. **Quantitative data** in community interventions usually involve the selection of precoded responses to questions set in survey format. Surveys are administered to carefully drawn samples that are often large and allow statistical manipulation of factors or responses. Alternatively, questionnaires are administered to participants before and at one or more points after an intervention to determine the impact of the intervention. **Qualitative data** are obtained from individual or group interviews, participant observation with extensive field notes, or examination of public records. Interviews are transcribed, and the words from transcripts, field notes, and public records subjected to an analysis that involves multiple rereading of the text and organization of contents into categories and themes. Qualitative data are more likely to reveal the broader context of an issue or situation and contribute to the depth of understanding, because they capture nuances and issues that the investigator may not have thought of previously. Researchers may start with the collection of qualitative data to inform them on the issues that should be included in the development of a structured questionnaire to use in the collection of quantitative data.

COLLECTING QUANTITATIVE DATA

A variety of ways to collect data are available, including **Internet surveys** such as Survey Monkey (www.surveymonkey.com), **telephone surveys**, **group interviews,** and **one-on-one face-to-face interviews**. All these methods have methodological limitations. Mail surveys typically have a very low response rate and require several follow-up mailings to people who do not respond to the initial mailing. When sending out a survey in the mail, a stamped self-addressed envelope should be included to facilitate returns. Self-administered questionnaires are relatively efficient, but require a certain level of literacy on the part of participants. When cost is taken into consideration, however, face-to-face interviews are the most expensive because they require staff time. Internet questionnaires are probably the least expensive.

The data collection method selected will depend on the resources available to the project, as well as the resources of the target population and the amount of time the target population is willing to spend providing the required information. The timing of the interview must be considered. Participants who are working or attending school may need to be interviewed during evening hours, whereas mothers of young children are generally not available before or directly after school or during mealtime. The interviewer must be mindful of the length of time passing during any interview. Face-to-face interviews can be longer than those administered via other methods, but it is wise to restrict the interview to about an hour to maintain good rapport with the respondent and obtain meaningful responses. The length of time that a respondent will sit still while talking to an interviewer also depends on the salience of the subject matter to the respondent and the skills of the interviewer.

Also important are the ability to recruit the target population, the population's skills, the training and skills of the staff, and the time and space available for data collection. Clearly, an **Internet survey** is not useful if the target population does not have access to computers. An Internet survey can be taken only by people who are computer-literate and may therefore miss populations like the elderly, who have more limited computer skills. Conversely, very limited financial resources available for data collection and a target population sophisticated in electronic communication such as high school or college students might make an Internet survey a good choice. Face-to-face interviews are costly if a large sample is required. Health care providers are usually not willing to spend much of their time completing such surveys, but might be willing to take part in a short phone interview. If this method is selected, be certain to make an appointment for the phone interview before the interview itself. A phone interview during the day will miss people who are working or in school, may require many call-backs, and will also leave out people who rely solely on cell phones. Rural populations living a considerable distance from each other might benefit from a telephone intervention preceded and followed by a telephone survey.

The location for a face-to-face interview must be considered. An intervention focusing on women who have young children may require space and staff for child care both during the data collection and the intervention. Determining the reproductive health needs of men may require a neutral community location, because men may not want to meet in a family planning clinic, which is viewed as feminine territory. Researchers may have to learn this information about their target population on a trial-and-error basis, adjusting data collection and intervention implementation protocols as necessary.

The types of data to be collected also depend on other factors such as the questions to be answered and the depth and detail needed about the impact of the intervention. The research question to be answered in the intervention will determine whether data collection consists of quantitative data, qualitative data, or both types. If minimal information about factors associated with a research question is needed, qualitative methods using individual or group interviews with open-ended questions will provide the necessary data. Using multiple methods of data collection is called **triangulation.** Use of multiple methods saves time and provides a greater depth of understanding about an issue; it also minimizes the limitations that are present in a single-method study design (Creswell & Clark, 2007). For example, it is helpful to get quantitative demographic information using a questionnaire about people *before* they begin their participation in a qualitative focus group. Conducting in-depth interviews with the respondents to a questionnaire provides a greater depth of understanding about specific issues while also allowing for a statistical analysis of the questionnaire's data.

Instrument Development

Quantitative data collection involves the use of structured **instruments** or **questionnaires** in which the questions and possible responses have been previously determined. Ideally, the questions in the instrument have been developed in previous research projects or identified through a literature search on interventions with the population and topic of interest. This process may be time-consuming, because many journals that publish intervention results are not able to make the instruments available. It may be possible to construct the items in the instrument from the results of the data analysis. Alternatively, writing to the lead author for permission to use the instrument is strongly suggested. It is worthwhile to spend time on identifying appropriate instruments *before* the start of the intervention. Such instruments have been found to be reliable by other researchers, and it is not necessary to determine whether the **psychometric properties** of the instrument are adequate. It may also be possible to adapt an instrument used on the topic of interest but with a different population. For example, a **pre- and post-survey** used with rural women in an intervention to increase physical activity may need some minor modifications to be used with urban African American women. Use of questions that have been developed and used by others is definitely encouraged.

If no appropriate instrument exists to use or adapt, it may be necessary to develop a new instrument. The material for such instruments is often developed from the results of preliminary unstructured interviews. There are several different types of questions that can be constructed in research instruments, including open- and closed-ended questions and forced-choice questions.

A **closed-ended question** forces a respondent to select an answer from among the alternative categories offered such as, "Did you eat fruit or vegetables at dinner last night?" Forcing a choice between possible responses can be helpful if answers in precise categories are required, such as the number of times in the past week people ate dinner out in a restaurant. Closed-ended questions are easier to deal with at the data entry stage (discussed later in this chapter). However, they have a potential limitation when used for sensitive topics such as drug use in which respondents may select the lowest frequency offered, knowing this to be a more socially desirable answer. The wording and language used in closed-ended questions should be understood in the same way by the researcher and the respondent or the results will not accurately describe what the researchers are seeking to discover. For example, when asked if they are "sexually active," some teens may interpret the wording of the question as asking about a variety of sexual activities, whereas others may think it means only vaginal intercourse. If the wording of a question can be interpreted in a variety of ways, the answers to the question will reflect this ambiguity, and the data collected will not be reliable.

The advantage of **open-ended questions** is that they do not force people to choose between a few responses, none of which may accurately reflect their choice. For example, if girls are asked which competitive sport they would most like to participate in and are given the choice of basketball, volleyball, or softball, those who prefer hockey or soccer would be missed. The disadvantage of open-ended questions is that they must be reviewed and coded after the interview has been completed, and this is a time-consuming task.

Forced-choice questions compel respondents to select among choices such as agree or disagree, or true or false. This certainly makes data entry and analysis easier; respondents may feel compelled to respond in ways that they believe are correct or socially desirable (such as "Yes, I always use condoms" or "No, I don't use drugs").

The number of choices must also be considered; a question like "Sexual activity among youth should be discouraged" does not allow for many gradations of opinion if only two choices are offered. An alternative format is to offer more choices in a **Likert-type response,** where four or five choices are provided, such as strongly agree, agree, neutral/not sure, disagree, or strongly disagree. Unfortunately, even this is not a perfect format because some authorities feel that Likert-type questions are not easily or accurately answered by members of many ethnic minority groups (Lee, Jones, Mineyama, & Zhang, 2002). Even given these problems, time and resource constraints may call for the development of a structured instrument. If this is the case, following are several general guidelines to keep in mind.

■   Always phrase the questions using language that most people can understand. Most authorities suggest that questionnaires should be written at a reading level no higher than sixth grade (Stommel & Wills, 2003). Reading level can be assessed in most word processing programs (in Microsoft Word, this function is available in Tools–Spelling & Grammar–Options).

■   Do not ask more than one question in a single item. For example, the phrasing, "Did you think that the information was clearly written and provided important information?" should be broken into two separate questions.

■   The order of questions can influence the responses because the way one question is worded can suggest an answer to the next question. For example, if asking about sensitive topics such as the consistency of condom use, people are more apt to change their answers if they see that answers to questions close in proximity (for example, "Did you use a condom the last time you had sexual intercourse?") are inconsistent. Answers to questions about risk behavior early in a questionnaire may influence later answers about risky sexual activity. Questions with related content generally tend to influence each other more if they are in close proximity.

■   Try not to ask questions that may be interpreted as invasive early on in an interview or a questionnaire, such as, "What was your income last year?" Start with questions that are easy to answer, like "How long have you lived in this community?" If you ask a question about income in a written survey, provide categories of income in check-off boxes. In a face-to-face interview, provide the participant with a card with letters next to different income levels and ask them which letter best describes their income (Creswell & Clark, 2007).

■   Keep the wording consistent throughout the questionnaire and between participants. Changing the wording may influence the answer.

■   Always leave categories open for no response, "don't know," "not applicable," and "other" categories for answers that do not fit other response categories. If very few answers fall into these categories, they can be ignored in the data analysis. If numerous answers fall into these categories, there are statistical methods for dealing with this problem.

■   Be aware of **respondent fatigue.** While there is no fixed maximum number of questions people are willing to answer, there is certainly an upper limit. Factors influencing length are the environment (fewer outside a supermarket, standing with a bag of groceries, more in a prearranged meeting in a comfortable room with refreshments available), the population (fewer with children or participants with short attention spans), and the topic (more if an area of concern).

▤   Lay out the questions so that participants can move easily from one question to the next without getting confused. Provide enough space between the lines to easily read the questions. Do not place a question on one page and its possible responses on another. Provide an introduction to the overall instrument and transition sentences to the different parts (such as "Now we would like to ask you a few questions about your health habits"). Be sure to add a statement such as, "Thank you for completing these questions" at the end, in a larger font than the rest of the document.

▤   To ensure that all staff members are meticulous in their collection methods, leave time in each week to meet and review the data that have been collected. For example, in open-ended interviews with different respondents, if it appears that respondents are using exactly the same words to answer a question, this may indicate that the interviewer is rephrasing responses rather than using the respondents' own wording. If this is the case, the data are contaminated and will need to be discarded.

Whether a previously used or newly developed instrument is selected, it is important that the instrument be have a pilot test to try out before being used in the field. Piloting the instrument will provide an idea of the flow of the questionnaire. With a previously used instrument, questions from another area of the country or the world may be misunderstood and need to be reformulated. Some questions may elicit almost the same response from everyone and should probably be tossed out because there is no variation in responses.

Collecting Follow-Up Data

To evaluate the success of a community intervention and see whether it has resulted in any change in attitudes or behavior, it is necessary to survey participants at the end of the program. Many researchers also select a study design that surveys participants a few weeks to months after the program to gauge whether changes have been sustained. Follow-up with the same respondents may be a challenge in communities where people move frequently or with populations anxious about being identified, such as substance users. To reinterview the same people over a period of time, it will be necessary to develop a tracking system in which all participants are asked at the end of the first interview to provide their locating data (name, address, phone numbers, and e-mail) and also some information about one or two people close to them who will know how to contact them if they move. This person may be a family member, a neighbor, or a best friend. Information about the tracking system should be kept in a file or database separate from other data. A record should be made of every attempted contact and a procedure established for the number and order of contacts that will be made (for example, initial phone call followed by e-mail, followed by letter, followed by house visit). The replacement of land phone lines by cell phones has made follow-up an even greater challenge, as there are no phone directories to provide this information. Do not minimize the importance of repeated attempts, as an 80 percent follow-up rate is far stronger than a 50 percent response rate (Kelly, Ahmed, Martinez, & Peralez-Dieckmann, 2007).

Sampling and Related Issues

Interviewing every individual in a community or population of interest is expensive, time-consuming, and unnecessary, given current statistical techniques. Including a **sample** or selection of part of the population in the evaluation or research design will generally provide the necessary information. A reliable sampling method is very important in understanding community values and attitudes before designing and implementing an intervention or arguing about the accuracy of an evaluation. Selecting a sample that gives everyone in the target population an equal chance of being selected substantially strengthens a study design, because it helps prevent the sample from being biased in a particular way. This is why the volunteer method is not relied on for recruitment into a sample. The goal is to develop a sampling method that is as representative of the entire population as possible. Once the sample has been selected, the participants must be randomly assigned to the intervention and a comparison group. The comparison group will be excluded from the intervention. Randomization occurs at the time of entry into a study for individuals or at the time of initiation of the intervention if working with institutions such as schools or sports clubs. These units of analysis can be systematically selected by a **randomization** procedure as simple as putting names in a hat or by assigning random numbers from a chart of random numbers, which can be found at the back of most introductory statistics books. Many situations do not allow for random assignment of individuals. For example, if the intervention is an addition to the school health curriculum, the classes within a grade can be randomly assigned to the intervention or comparison group, even though the individual students may not be assigned to the intervention or comparison group.

A **convenience sample** is one that works with the available participants or other units of analysis—for example, the patients in the waiting room of a local clinic or two churches with which the researcher is familiar. This type of sample may be all that is possible and is generally very adequate for preliminary studies. A **snowball sample,** also known as a respondent-driven sample, starts with a small group of participants who are part of a larger network with which they share information about the study. The initial participants are asked to provide names of friends or coworkers who share the particular network. This type of strategy works well with hard-to-reach populations such as caretakers in an immigrant community or sex workers.

Sample size is something that must be considered before attempting a statistical analysis of the data. The sample must be large enough to provide adequate statistical **power** to show statistically significant results. With primary data, the size of the sample will ultimately depend on the available resources. The more participants in a program or surveyed in any sample, the greater the cost. It is possible to do a **descriptive analysis** or **cross-tabulations** with a relatively small sample. However, the results will not be statistically meaningful if the sample size is below twenty-five (unless a feasibility or **pilot study** is being conducted). For information about sampling and sample size, consult a standard statistics book.

Care must be taken to ensure that recruitment does not result in a sample that skews the results. For example, interviewing only volunteers may result in a sample made up of individuals from the target population who have extra time on their hands or who have a particular ax to grind. Such a sample will also result in missing information from a whole segment of the community that does not have the time or inclination to volunteer. **Facilitators** such as travel funds or child care arrangements can help increase the breadth of the sample pool and thus have the potential of reducing bias, especially if it is possible to pay for people's time and travel.

COLLECTING QUALITATIVE DATA

Qualitative data can be gathered in a variety of ways, including observation, interviews with key informants, in-depth or unstructured interviewing, and focus groups. **Observational data** are collected by an observer who carefully notes the details of events transpiring over a specific period of time or during an occasion. This method is useful in determining how to reach a target population and might be used to identify who seems to be part of the "in crowd" in a school class and who seems to be more on the fringe. An observer should be as unobtrusive as possible so that her presence does not change the situation, as people being observed may adjust their behavior if it becomes obvious that they are being watched. For example, bullying in a school yard may cease if the pupils involved think that they are being observed by an adult.

Types of Interviews

Interviewing key informants can be done using open-ended questions or with a more **structured interview guide. Key informants** are people who represent some segments of the larger community, such as elected officials or their staff, chairs of a tenants committee, health care providers, or church leaders. Key informants can provide information about how a community is likely to react to interventions about sensitive issues such as sexual activity or drug use, what local needs are, and whether a specific intervention has made an impact on the target population. Open-ended questions are phrased in a neutral manner such as, "How do you think teachers responded to the violence prevention training?" or "What do you think should be done about the high rate of adolescent pregnancy in this community?" A structured interview guide is a series of questions determined in advance that the interviewer will return to as the discussion wanders from topic to topic. The questions do not have to be asked in order; rather, they serve as a checklist to ensure that the interviewer has covered all the topics.

In-depth interviewing or an unstructured interview is more like an open-ended discussion about a topic in which the respondent may take the discussion into areas not previously envisioned by the interviewer. Since the interviewer does not know in advance all the questions that are pertinent to a topic, allowing a discussion to flow into unanticipated areas is likely to yield useful information. In an unstructured or in-depth interview the interviewer must learn to **probe** respondents for more information if it appears that aspects of the issue are not covered completely. An interviewer guide will suggest helpful probes on specific issues, and a few **follow-up questions** are useful when a simple yes-or-no answer will not suffice.

Group Interviews

A **focus group** interview is conducted with a small group of people (six to twelve) to explore the issues of interest. This method has been used for many years by market researchers to assess consumer attitudes toward a product. Data derived from focus group discussions often lead to new ideas and concepts. Since the participants generally share some aspect of the topic under discussion, they are able to build on each other's statements or challenge each other on features of their shared cultures with which the researcher may not be familiar. Members of the group may be selected because they represent the community or that portion of the community that has been targeted. Or they may be members of the target community who are known to be articulate or knowledgeable about the topic of interest. Questions for the interview in the form of a **discussion guide** are developed prior to the focus group meeting. A facilitator conducts the meeting and is responsible for making certain that all the questions are covered, that no one dominates the discussion, and that all members of the focus group are heard from. One or two people from the research team should take careful notes of the discussion to determine who made specific points. Frequently, a tape recorder is used to record the discussion, but it can be difficult to transcribe all the specific comments. Even if the recording is not transcribed, it is very useful to check with written notes. The assembled group should be asked for permission to record their conversation. Once the recording is started, the presence of a tape recorder is soon forgotten.

Before the discussion begins, it is essential for the subsequent analysis that the note taker develop a notation system that will indicate who said what. For example, an identification number can be given to each discussion member and used to anonymously identify each individual. The numbers can be placed on a chart of participants in the room so that the speakers can easily be identified by number. The note taker should record the first few words of speakers according to their number on the chart. This record can be added into the transcribed tapes and will enable the data analyst to tell if just one or two people are responding or if opinions come from a larger number of group members. Also included in the meeting notes should be a legend detailing the demographic characteristics of each of the participants (age, education, occupation, ethnicity, and so forth). Noting some identifying characteristic (such as crazy red shirt or laughing older man) will help visualize the taped data as it is transcribed as well as fully describe the participants of the group. It is helpful to start the meeting with an easy warm-up question like "What was your favorite vacation?" or "If you could be an animal, what animal would you be, and why?" It helps the group spirit if snacks are provided before the focus group meeting gets going. As a rule of thumb, the entire meeting should not last more than one and a half to two hours. It is wise to invite ten to twelve people if a group of eight is desired, because not everyone who was asked to participate will show up.

Managing Qualitative Data

Sample size for qualitative data is determined differently than that of quantitative data. **Saturation**—the point at which no new information is being collected or the information being gathered becomes repetitive—is used as a guide for an adequate sample. For straightforward questions, a rule of thumb of twenty to twenty-five respondents is generally adequate (Creswell, 1998).

The notes and audiotapes from interview data should be transcribed as soon as possible after collection. To facilitate transcription of audiotapes, purchase an inexpensive foot pedal that can be attached to the tape recorder. Using this foot control to start, stop, and reverse the tape allows the transcriber's hands to remain on the keyboard and greatly speeds transcription. As a rule of thumb, it takes three to four hours to transcribe an hour-long interview or focus group.

The data collected by qualitative methods tend to be voluminous and must be coded by theme to make them more accessible and understandable to others. This can be done by hand or using a computer program specifically designed for this task such as NUD*IST or ATLAS.ti. The written text is carefully read, and repeated patterns of responses are assigned codes as themes seem to emerge. These themes become the basis of findings from the data (Lofland & Lofland, 1995). When you are coding by hand, it is preferable to have several people read through the data to pick out common themes, with differences of opinions being discussed until resolution is reached.

AFTER DATA COLLECTION

As surveys are turned in, they should be placed in a common envelope or bin that a member of the research team will watch carefully. Consent forms or locator forms should be placed in a different envelope. If the event is held during evening hours or at several locations, make arrangements to have all data returned to the office as soon as possible—the next day at the latest. In the office, data should be kept in a locked cabinet, with locator data kept in a separate file from the data itself.

After collection, data are entered into a database so that it is possible to see how the answers to questions differ among groups such as males and females or older and younger members. Most researchers use either Excel, available in Microsoft Office packages, or SPSS, a user-friendly statistical program that offers a less expensive student version available from university bookstores or the manufacturer. The decisions about how data will be entered and how the analysis will proceed should be finalized before beginning data collection. This will avoid situations like having data collected from fifty participants, only to find that the necessary software for analysis is not available on any computer.

To facilitate data entry, it is a good idea to **precode** the responses, that is, to include the data entry codes on the survey form itself. This allows each response to be easily entered into the computer program. See Exhibit 6.1 for an example.

EXHIBIT 6.1 **Sample survey with data entry codes**

1. What is your gender?
   _____male (1)
   _____female (2)
2. What is your educational level?
   _____less than high school diploma (1)
   _____some college (2)
   _____college graduate (3)
   _____graduate degree (4)
How much do you agree or disagree with the following statements?

	STRONGLY AGREE (1)	AGREE (2)	NEITHER AGREE OR DISAGREE (3)	DISAGREE (4)	STRONGLY DISAGREE (5)
3. Men are better leaders than women					
4. It is more important for boys to graduate from college than for girls					
5. It is worse for girls to get into fights than for boys					

After each data entry session, be sure that the data are backed up on another system. When all the data are entered, a check for accuracy should be conducted. One way to do this is to pull every tenth survey and, with someone who has not done the data entry, compare the responses on the survey with the codes typed into the database.

If the error rate is higher than 10 percent, it will be necessary to go back and check that each of the surveys has been accurately entered. If resources are available, it is possible to avoid the data input process by having responses recorded directly onto a precoded questionnaire printed on special paper that can be scanned directly into a computer. There are also handheld computers on which respondents can enter their answers, which then can be directly downloaded onto a computer at the end of the day. When deciding on which data entry system to select, remember that while questionnaires that can be directly scanned into the computer or handheld computers may seem expensive, data entry is time-consuming and can be costly.

After quantitative data are entered, they must be cleaned. This entails reviewing all the data and detecting and deleting responses that have been entered inaccurately or erroneously. A part of this process is checking for **outliers**—values that are outside the expected range of values, such as age sixty-five on a survey of adolescents. A second check can be done for codes that are not possible. Both of these checks can be easily done by running a frequency distribution and examining the results.

Remember that new variables will have to be created to provide aggregate scores for items like knowledge and attitudes. This is done by using the computer program to add together all the related knowledge or attitude items into a **scale** and giving the resultant variable a new name. For example, in Exhibit 6.1, above question, there should be a final variable that might be called "Attitudes About Women" and would be the sum of questions 3, 4, and 5. As data are being entered, be sure that a backup system is in place. At this point, the data are finally ready for statistical analysis. Statistics consist of two basic types: descriptive and inferential. Descriptive statistics describe a population by summarizing the relevant data into proportions (percentages), measures of central tendency (mean, median, and mode), measures of dispersion (variance, standard deviation, and range), and correlation coefficients (used to show relationships between two variables). Inferential statistics are used to draw inferences about a population from a data sample. If the sample size is not large enough to be representative of the population, inferential statistics may not be the most effective choice. At the very least, however, a descriptive analysis should be done because it provides an accurate way to describe the collected data. For a more in-depth discussion of descriptive and inferential statistics, refer to an introductory statistics book such as Mirkin (2005) or Munro (2005).

SUMMARY

This chapter provided the basic information necessary for understanding data: what it is, where to get it, when to collect it, how to use it, and who will use it. In addition to providing a general discussion about data, this chapter covered the various quantitative and qualitative techniques that practitioners use when planning, implementing, and evaluating community-based interventions.

KEY TERMS

Closed-ended question
Convenience sample
Data
Data processing
Data set
Descriptive analysis or cross-tabulations
Discussion guide
Facilitators
Focus group
Follow-up question
Forced-choice question
Group interview
Instruments
Internet survey
Key informant
Large data sets
Likert-type response
Observational data
One-on-one face-to-face interview
Open-ended question
Outlier
Pilot study

Power
Pre- and post-survey
Precode
Primary data
Probe
Psychometric properties
Qualitative data
Quantitative data
Questionnaire
Randomization
Respondent fatigue
Sample
Sample size
Saturation
Scale
Secondary data
Snowball sample (also known as a respondent-driven sample)
Structured interview guide
Telephone surveys
Triangulation
Variable

ACTIVITIES

1. Describe a specific target population for whom an Internet-based survey would be appropriate. Why do you think it would work with this group? What research and/or statistics support your claim?

2. From your professional experience and the literature you have read, identify a target population for a health intervention and a question that might be answered through a community-based health intervention. Which method is most appropriate to answer the question? Why?

3. Identify a questionnaire that has been used to collect information about a health topic in which you are interested. Discuss the ways in which the instrument is useful. Critique the questionnaire. Precode at least fifteen of the questions and pilot-test the questionnaire with five members of your target population. Share your findings.

DISCUSSION QUESTIONS

1. You have been asked to prepare a discussion guide and conduct a focus group of teenage girls on strategies to address dating violence.

   a. What type(s) of data are you collecting?

   b. What are some important steps that must be taken to accomplish these tasks?

   c. Cite possible challenges you might face while undertaking this exercise.

   d. Explain how you plan to overcome these challenges.

2. Examine the data on the National Center for Health Statistics web site (www.cdc .gov/nchs) and discuss which features you find most useful and which features you find least useful.

PART

3

WORKING THROUGH
THE INTERVENTION

ASSESSING COMMUNITY NEEDS

LEARNING OBJECTIVES

- Understand the rationale for a community assessment
- Implement the steps necessary for conducting a community assessment
- Become familiar with the options available for sharing the results of an assessment with community partners and other interested stakeholders

OVERVIEW

This chapter covers the rationale for and the practical components of a community assessment. Different approaches to working with community members and disseminating assessment findings are also presented.

BASIC COMPONENTS OF A COMMUNITY ASSESSMENT

A **community assessment** provides practitioners and stakeholders who are planning an intervention with a road map that helps them decide what direction to take, what intervention goals to focus on, and what **objectives** are necessary to reach the goal or desired end point (outcomes). Community assessments generally include five components: formulating guiding questions, selecting assessment type, collecting data, analyzing data, and identifying priority needs and service gaps (Academy for Educational Development, 1994). This information can be used to demonstrate to funding agencies that a particular project or intervention warrants financial support (Petersen & Alexander, 2001; Soriano, 1995). A community assessment informs the development of an intervention by revealing unmet health needs within a community. For interventions that are already underway, community assessments provide a means to gauge how well the intervention elements have been achieved and what needs to be reworked or discontinued to reach stated objectives. For projects that have already been funded, information gathered from a community assessment can help justify and build a case for obtaining further funding (Petersen & Alexander, 2001; Soriano, 1995).

Connecting with Stakeholders

The first step in conducting a community assessment is to organize the available resources and time needed to become familiar with as many aspects of the community as possible. Begin by connecting with key community members or stakeholders. **Stakeholders** are community "insiders" who have a vested interest in the success of an implemented intervention. Examples of potential stakeholders are decision makers within service provision agencies (such as health care clinics, schools, churches, and businesses) and individuals who might find the information useful for their own work. Other potential stakeholders include influential sources close to individuals who use the developed services including family members, clergy members, and informal community leaders such as the chair of a tenants association. Stakeholders also include formal groups that are working within the community, such as community partnerships and community advisory boards.

Developing a **working group** consisting of stakeholders and other community members can strengthen the communication between the practitioner and the target group. Stakeholders can provide practitioners with details about the community that are unavailable elsewhere. They can open doors for practitioners and help them connect with others who play influential roles within the community. Such connections can help familiarize practitioners with the terrain of the community's past. They can provide insights into potential impediments to community assessments such as individuals or groups who might challenge the assessment process. Teaming up with stakeholders from the start provides practitioners a way to garner their ideas and feedback throughout the assessment process. This involvement not only helps ensure the success of the community assessment, but also increases the chances of community support when the intervention is implemented after the assessment is completed.

Formulating Guiding Questions

Once community support seems assured, the community assessment can begin. The first step is to develop a set of questions that describe the population and the problem that will be addressed in an ideal intervention. Guiding questions might include, What is the problem? Who is the affected community? Who is the target population? What issues are being faced by this population? What resources are available to this population? While these questions are broad at first, it is important to note that they will become more specific as the community assessment progresses.

Types of Assessments

The next step is to choose the type of assessment that will be conducted. In practice, three distinct approaches to conducting a community assessment have emerged. The first is a **needs assessment,** an assessment approach that identifies and reports on the needs, problems, and deficiencies of an affected community (Petersen & Alexander, 2001). The second approach is a **capacity assessment,** an assessment approach that identifies actual or potential resources or assets that can ameliorate community problems (Gilmore & Campbell, 2005). Four types of resources are likely to positively affect community problems, including:

- **Individual resources,** such as person(s)' specific skills, past involvement in community-based work, and individual readiness to engage in and contribute to changing the health status of the community

- **Institutional resources,** including formal institutions such as schools, libraries, parks, police stations, hospitals, colleges, universities, and informal institutions such as community associations, faith-based groups, or any volunteer group that might be able to participate in and contribute to changing the health status of the community

- **Physical structures** such as land, buildings, transportation, established infrastructure, and natural resources that could contribute to changing the health status of the community

- **Economic assets,** including businesses or informal economic exchanges such as barter relationships that can influence the health status of the community (Kretzmann & McKnight, 1993)

A third community assessment approach studies both the needs and strengths of a community. The needs assessment and the capacity assessment each provide only a partial snapshot of the community; a more comprehensive picture can be drawn by assessing both (W. K. Kellogg Foundation, 2004). Thus, this chapter will focus on community assessments that explore both community needs and strengths. The wider lens of the community assessment approach provides a more accurate view and produces more effective interventions.

Collecting Data

With the assessment type selected, the practitioner begins to select the data sources that will be consulted and the assessment methods that will be used to collect the data. It is important to keep in mind that the type of data collected and the assessment methods employed are highly dependent on the project's available resources (such as time and money). Usual data sources consist of **preexisting data** (derived from secondary sources) and **community input** (gathered through primary sources). Preexisting sets of information, or secondary data sources, usually provide epidemiological data. In contrast, community input or data generated through primary data collection methods provide information from members of the community, service providers, and others who are knowledgeable about both the health needs and the primary health concerns of the community.

Preexisting Data

One job for those engaged in a community assessment is the location of existing data relevant to the state, city, and neighborhood that can be significant for the community assessment. In addition to large national data sets, using state, city, and neighborhood data allows the practitioner to determine how the health of the target population compares to the health of other populations in different geographic areas of comparable size and demographics. Such data enable practitioners to determine how the target population's health compares to the overall health of the city, state, and nation in which it is located. Many agencies, such as state and city health departments, collect and make available data on health services and health-related statistics.

Local or state public agencies such as police departments, libraries, hospitals, and clinics can also be resources for a variety of secondary source data. For instance, hospital patient records can provide insight into the occurrence rates of a particular health problem. Hospital records include medical histories, clinical reports, prescribed treatments and procedures, and discharge summaries, all of which can be used to assess items like patterns of emergency room use over a given period of time. Keep in mind, however, that regulations such as the Health Insurance Portability and Accountability Act (HIPAA) will influence the availability of these types of records. To protect patient confidentiality, these records are very hard to access unless all identifying information has been expunged from them. More on this subject is discussed in Chapter Three.

University departmental research projects that collect data on community studies or other community-related projects can also be consulted as another source of secondary data information. Published research studies can provide information that can increase understanding of the target community or a community that is similar in key aspects (such as immigrant population, health problems, or resources).

Information or data that are not directly related to health give the practitioner a more robust understanding of the target community. Such sources include economic and industrial information from the local chamber of commerce or elementary or high school attendance records. Local community boards that collect and provide data on sociodemographics, homeowners, renters, and employment rates can also add significant perspectives to the community assessment. Newspaper and community newsletter information on community-related news items, employment opportunities, and editorials can shed light on local current events and issues and their relevance to the community assessment.

Analyzing Data

Once the secondary and primary data have been collected, the information needs to be analyzed. Initially, a comparison of the target community's data with other communities in the nation—especially those demographically similar in size and income levels—can be helpful. This comparison will not provide definitive answers, but it can estimate average trends and lend perspective to the community assessment. The next step, a triangulation analysis of both the quantitative and qualitative data, will provide a richer picture of the target community. (This more formal approach to analyzing the collected material is discussed in Chapter Six.)

STRENGTHENING YOUR FINDINGS

While data collected through secondary sources can provide critical insights, such information may not be sufficient to ensure that the practitioner's assumptions are valid about the community's wants, needs, and willingness to act. Therefore, combining primary data collected from people living and working in the community with secondary data provides a more accurate picture of community members' experiences. Primary data consist of information that is collected for an express purpose through surveys, focus groups, and independent observations. (For information on surveys and focus groups, see Chapter Six.)

Community Input

Independent observations are also known as **windshield surveys** or **mapping** exercises. They involve the practitioner traveling around the community either by foot or by car to create an inventory of visual factors or barriers that facilitate or inhibit healthy behaviors. This information helps the practitioner locate not only existing resources that can ameliorate identified health problems but also where gaps in services may lie. The types of questions a practitioner may ask while visually exploring the community can include: What are the geographic or commercial boundaries of the community?

What kind of housing is available in the community (whether apartments, multifamily dwellings, or high-rises)? What types of organizations provide services to residents (organizations, hospitals, child care services, and so forth)? What types of parks or open spaces exist in the community? What kinds of stores and commercial facilities can residents shop at (such as grocery, liquor, or big-box stores)? What kinds of community gathering spots are there (senior centers or youth camps, for instance)? Are there private or public schools in the community? How do residents travel within and out of the community? Is the community safe (is there evidence of gang-related activity or a police presence)? For more information on conducting a mapping exercise, see Warren and Warren (1984) or visit www.arlingtonva.us/Departments/HumanServices/PublicHealth/MAPP/page60408.aspx.

Identifying Priority Needs and Service Gaps

After the data have been analyzed, the next step entails putting these identified needs into a form that is useful for determining whether resources already exist in the community that can address these needs.

Prioritizing the results of a community assessment is a decision-making process whereby steps are taken to arrange assessment findings into categories ranging from "most pressing health need" to "least pressing health need" (Brownson, Baker, Leet, & Gillespie, 2003; Timmreck, 2003). Stakeholders should be involved in prioritizing assessment findings to ensure that decisions reflect the opinions held by those within the community. If stakeholders are not involved, practitioners run the risk of inaccurately gauging community responsiveness. For example, in an East Coast city, an initial analysis of assessment data collected by planners from the city health department revealed that childhood asthma and lead poisoning rates were proportionally higher in certain neighborhoods and constituted a pressing health problem. These findings, if taken alone, would suggest that action should be taken to ameliorate the environmental conditions creating these health issues. However, a previously formed work group of community members and local organizational representatives reported to health department employees that inadequate sanitation and pest control problems presented a greater concern. Contrary to initial analysis, community stakeholders were not primarily interested in services that addressed asthma and lead poisoning because they felt rat infestations and subsequent rat bites warranted more immediate attention. Using the information gathered from engaged stakeholders, the advisory group and health department employees decided that city assistance should first focus on sanitation and pest control interventions and then address other health problems in the community.

This account demonstrates that working with interested stakeholders is important in coming to agreement about the order of priority of unmet needs found in a community assessment. Such agreement between the research team and stakeholders increases the odds that community leaders and the larger community will welcome the intervention, rather than view it as imposed on them by outsiders.

To fully participate in the decision-making process that determines which of the community assessment findings should be initially addressed, everyone involved should be able to understand and use the assessment data. The data should be organized and explained in a manner that is clear and easily understood by both professionals and laypeople. Typically, reports and oral presentations are used to communicate findings. Both approaches benefit from the use of visual aids to facilitate the clear and well-organized presentation of findings. For instance, visual presentations such as bar graphs, line graphs, and pie graphs created through computer spreadsheet programs (such as Excel) offer a pictorial view of the community assessment data.

Some specific techniques are helpful in organizing the discussions and processes of group meetings. A good **moderator** or **facilitator** can balance participation and also assure that the desired outcomes of the meeting are met. An ideal choice is someone who is trusted by participants but not necessarily one of the key stakeholders. Having a prepared agenda helps with the organization of content. Determine whether decisions will be made by majority vote or if group consensus will be required. Use the time together to schedule the next meeting before the group breaks up.

Another strategy designed to stimulate group feedback is the **nominal group technique**, a series of brainstorming exercises designed to encourage members to voice their opinions, examine the opinions of others, and reach a group consensus on prioritizing the assessment findings (Van de Ven & Delbecq, 1971). The **basic priority rating system** involves asking group members to rank assessment findings based on three components: the size of the problem, the seriousness of the problem, and the estimated effectiveness of the solution (Hanlon, 1973). The highest-ranked problem found in the assessment would receive priority within the planning process. Details on these techniques are available in community assessment textbooks (for example, Gilmore & Campbell, 2005; Simons-Morton, Greene, & Gottlieb, 1995; Vilnius & Dandoy, 1990).

The creation of a work group that includes engaged stakeholders throughout all stages of the community assessment provides a venue whereby assessment findings can be presented and discussed with stakeholders. The feedback from this group can guide and shape planning efforts. While work groups can operate in various ways, the creation and functioning of the group is essential to the success of the health practitioner's interface with the community.

Identifying Services and Other Resources

After prioritizing health needs, practitioners must determine whether resources exist to address these problems. Stakeholders are the most useful source for learning about currently available resources, as they are directly involved with, affected by, and aware of services within the community. One way to learn what services organizations offer community residents is to visit with an agency's administrator or program coordinator and ask directly about their resources and services. This is a time-consuming process, however, so an alternative strategy is to talk to employees who do case management or social work for community organizations. These individuals spend a great deal of time linking clients to appropriate health and social services. Many will have created or used some form of a community resource directory. Government agencies such as health departments regularly identify and categorize existing services into resource directories that are often available via telephone or the Internet. Other community features such as transportation, parks, and walking trails can be identified through observation. Of course, the Internet can also be used to locate the community services that are available to the target population.

If services are found to be unavailable to address an identified health concern, this suggests an area where a new intervention might be developed (see Chapter Eight). However, if services do exist, the next step is to assess why the target population is not using them. For instance, organizations that serve the elderly may fail to attract local seniors if the community has no viable transportation. Practitioners can draw on the community assessment findings for assistance in determining where services can be enhanced. Stakeholders can also provide insights into the factors that may be hindering individuals from accessing community resources.

SUMMARY

The identification of pressing health needs within a community is best done through a systematic community assessment. The specific design of a community assessment depends on existing and available resources. The process uses both preexisting data and community input to determine and prioritize needs. Community involvement contributes greatly to the success of an assessment and establishes relationships for a future intervention based on the outcomes.

KEY TERMS

Basic priority rating system

Capacity assessment

Community assessment

Community input

Economic assets

Individual resources

Institutional resources

Moderator or facilitator

Needs assessment

Nominal group technique

Objectives

Physical structures

Preexisting data

Stakeholders

Windshield surveys or mapping

Working group

ACTIVITIES

1. Community assessments occasionally must be conducted quickly and without sufficient time to research anything beyond a review of statistics and relevant literature.

Imagine you are a program administrator for a national health organization. On Monday, you learn there is a request for proposals addressing the exact issues your organization focuses on daily, which also happen to be important to you as a student. The application is due on Friday. Think about what you know about a given population or health problem and how you would capture this information and make a compelling case for funding an ideal intervention to address a problem with which you are familiar.

    a.   What is the problem?

    b.   Who is affected?

    c.   Who is the target population? How old are they? Where do they live?

    d.   What else do you know about the problem or the population?

2. Think about the most relevant data sources you might draw on to further describe the population and the problem. What are they, and why do you think they would help build your case?

3. Conduct a search for literature describing the problem affecting the specific population you selected. Identify two relevant articles to describe the health problems facing your population of interest. Remember: the goal is not to locate every article ever written, but rather to read through the more relevant literature and report on the most salient and relevant articles.

DISCUSSION QUESTIONS

Consider the following two community scenarios and discuss your answers.

Community Scenario 1: Description of an Urban Community

You are assessing an economically depressed semiurban community of about 250,000 people. You begin by conducting a windshield survey in which you drive around the area and record your impressions and the apparent resources and deficiencies. In the main-street downtown area, you see the following:

- Several ethnic restaurants, two fast-food restaurants, and a diner

- A used furniture store, hardware store, three women's clothing shops, used bookstore, and stationery store

- Post office and town hall

- Two bars

- Movie theater showing two first-run films

- Local newspaper office

Across from the movie theater is a small park with a few benches and a World War II memorial. On the main highway coming into town, there is a big-box store, a large supermarket, and a small mall with several chain restaurants, a shoe store, a pizza restaurant, a coffee bar, and a dollar store.

While driving around town for an hour or two, you also notice the following:

- Ten churches, three of which are operating food banks

- One general hospital and one Catholic hospital

- Three community clinics, a family planning clinic, six physician practices, and three dental offices

- Police department, fire department, and county health department

- One community college, three high schools, five middle schools, eight elementary schools, and one parochial elementary school

- One soup kitchen

- Four supermarkets and six small markets

- A crisis pregnancy center

If the secondary data sources you have been examining suggest that adolescent pregnancy is a problem in this community, where would you go to gather first-hand or primary information about the problem? What kinds of questions would you ask?

Where would you go if the primary data sources suggested that childhood asthma is a problem? Discuss how your answer to the preceding question differs from this one.

Community Scenario 2: Description of a Nonurban Community

You are assessing a rural town with a population of about twelve thousand people. The economic base of the town is farming and a small manufacturing plant. You begin by conducting a windshield survey in which you drive around the area and record your impressions of the apparent resources and deficiencies. In the main-street downtown area, you see the following:

- Municipal building

- Grange

- Library

- Three antique stores

- Two banks

- One physician practice, one law practice, and one dental office

- Auto supply store

On the road leading into town are two motels, a supermarket, two banks, a gas station, a chain drugstore, a car dealership, five different chain fast-food restaurants, a bowling alley, a hospital, and a big-box store.

While driving around town for an hour or two, you also notice the following:

- Five churches, one of which is operating a food pantry

- Police department, fire department, and county health department

- One community college, one high school, two middle schools, and four elementary schools

- Three small markets

- A crisis pregnancy center

If the secondary data sources you have been examining suggest that underage drinking and driving is a problem in this community, where would you go to gather first-hand or primary information about the problem? What types of questions would you ask?

Where would you go if the primary data sources suggested that cardiovascular disease had a disproportionate impact on the death rate in this community? How does your answer to the preceding question differ?

CHAPTER

8

PLANNING A COMMUNITY-BASED INTERVENTION

LEARNING OBJECTIVES

- Review resources for identifying possible health interventions
- Understand the importance of intervention fidelity
- Describe the steps involved in the development of a logic model

OVERVIEW

This chapter describes how to use results of a community health assessment to view the health problems in the target population and identify the resources that can potentially be used to address problems. Content will include the issues, steps, and resources that must be considered when planning a community-based health intervention and the structure that must be in place to maximize its likelihood of success.

■ ■ ■

The goal of every community-based health intervention is to address an unmet health need that has been identified by stakeholders and the practitioners following a community assessment. Addressing this health need will be the **overall goal** of an intervention. Developing an overall goal generally begins with stating the problem in broad terms such as reducing teen pregnancy, preventing falls among the elderly, or improving women's cardiovascular health. The **problem statement** also contains information about the specific population, such as:

■ To reduce the number of pregnancies among students in the Middletown High School District

■ To prevent falls among residents of the Center Senior Apartments

■ To improve the cardiovascular health of African American women in Smithville

INTERVENTION CONTENT AND FORMAT

In considering any community health problem such as the three preceding examples, a variety of approaches can be applied. Before deciding on an approach, it is necessary to examine existing research findings on the problem to select an intervention and develop effective objectives. For instance:

■ Several different approaches can be used to address the identified problem of adolescent pregnancy. Some evidence-based studies show that girls who drop out of school are at a higher risk of experiencing an unplanned pregnancy (Manlove, 1998). Other studies show that many teens experience unplanned pregnancies because they fail to use contraceptives or use them inconsistently (Mensch & Kandel, 1992). Evidence is also available to suggest that adolescent girls who participate in organized sports have lower rates of sexual risk behaviors and pregnancy (Miller, Sabo, Farrell, Barnes, & Melnick, 1998).

■ Another example is the variety of ways that the problem of preventing falls in the elderly can be addressed. Evidence is available showing that falls can be reduced by interventions such as home assessments to check for safety risks or installation of grab bars next to toilets and showers (Newton, 2006).

■ A final example suggesting multiple ways to address a health problem is the third problem statement in the preceding section on improving cardiovascular health. Successful interventions have been found with content that increases physical activity through walking or dance programs, while others have addressed this problem through interventions that change eating habits (Flores, 1995; Murphy, Nevill, Neville, Biddle, & Hardman, 2002).

Library research in the form of a background literature review is critical at this early stage of the planning. Without adequate research, the practitioner or researcher may inadvertently attempt intervention projects that have been tested and possibly failed in other locations. It is not necessary to reinvent the wheel. The **scientific literature** is rich with examples of developed interventions that have been rigorously assessed for their intervention effectiveness. Because a wealth of information is available, practitioners should research what others in the field are doing before settling on a particular programmatic approach. In particular, approaches that have demonstrated positive effects within the larger population of interest should be identified.

Examine Relevant Databases

Identifying research-based interventions involves an examination of databases and electronic tools that organize research information. A number of computer databases provide field-specific scientific literature including:

PubMed is a database developed by the National Library of Medicine. It provides access to over 4,000 journals, including literature relevant to community health, from any computer with Internet access.

The Cumulative Index to Nursing and Allied Health Literature **(CINAHL)** offers access to a variety of journals and other resources that are relevant to public health. This database references issues from 1937 to the present.

EMBASE indexes more than 3,500 international journals and covers a wide variety of topics including public health, health policy and management, occupational health, and environmental health.

The **Global Health Database** offers resources related to human health and disease, including information on communicable diseases, tropical diseases, parasitic diseases, human nutrition, community and public health, and medicinal and poisonous plants.

The **Web of Science** (also known as the Science Citation Index) consists of seven databases that offer access to information from numerous scientific disciplines, including medicine and public health.

In all these sources, searches can be done by person, place, or topic, as well as cited reference searching. All citation indexes (science, social sciences, and humanities) can be searched simultaneously. For those unfamiliar with electronic literature searching, the PubMed web site provides a good tutorial (www.ncbi.nlm.nih.gov/pubmed). Reference librarians are also an excellent resource for search assistance.

Be aware that searching indexed databases is not the same as conducting Internet searches. Typing in multiple terms such as *pregnancy, adolescent,* and *interventions* will not be successful. Instead, each of these terms is searched separately and then connectors known as **Boolean operators** are used to focus or connect the search terms. The three Boolean operators are *AND, OR,* and *NOT.* Using AND narrows a search, using OR broadens a search, and using NOT excludes words from the search. For more information on Boolean operators, visit Information Retrieval Education Resources at http://ir.exp.sis.pitt.edu/res2/view.php?rid=85.

Inclusion of the terms *meta-analysis* or *review article* in a search will often identify an article that reviews all the major interventions in, or what is currently known about, a target area. Limiting to a specific time period, such as the past ten years, is useful when a search turns up hundreds or thousands of articles.

In addition to academic literature searches, an Internet search will identify web sites with information about interventions, many with considerable detail. For example:

■ The **Community Guide** is a CDC-sponsored initiative that reviews and makes recommendations about evidence-based interventions on a wide variety of health topics (www.thecommunityguide.org).

■ The **Cochrane Review** describes interventions on many topics in terms of the evidence of their strengths (www.cochrane.org/reviews).

■ **Health-Evidence.ca,** funded by the Canadian Institutes of Health Research, provides access to an online registry of systematically reviewed public health and health promotion interventions (http://health-evidence.ca).

■ The **National Guideline Clearinghouse,** developed by the Agency for Healthcare Research and Quality, gives users access to a comprehensive database of evidence-based practice guidelines (www.guidelines.gov).

■ **Public Health Partners** provides access to public health journals, newsletters, and reports from government and community agencies (http://phpartners.org/guide.html).

■ **Google Scholar** can identify abstracts of articles that are relevant to searched topics, although the articles themselves must be purchased (http://scholar.google.com).

Forums and Conferences

Forums that are regularly used by professionals, such as conferences, list-servs, and newsletters, are another source for information on interventions. These forums provide a venue where professionals can share project findings and lessons learned with others. For example, many professionals present their work at local, state, and national conferences to highlight their intervention's profile and get feedback from peers on their work. Conference web sites often contain intervention information and web links to many topic-specific projects and their organizers.

Networking with people who have personal and professional experience in a particular area of public health is extremely valuable. Initiate discussions with colleagues who are working in your target public health area. Check with the local and state health departments to identify staff members who are familiar with the health problem of interest. Private foundations and state or federal granting agencies may fund interventions addressing the target health issue.

Such a thorough review of the scientific literature for effective strategies can familiarize the researcher with the strategies that have been used to address health problems in other communities. This knowledge can save resources of time, money, and effort.

Consider All Options

Interventions that address the identified community health problem should replicate a previous line of effective research. The selected intervention must also be acceptable to the targeted community. For example, the researcher might know that an intervention to increase access to contraceptives for adolescents is not going to garner support among key stakeholders in the Middletown community, no matter what the evidence-based literature might suggest. However, other options identified in the literature to address the overall aim that could be acceptable to the community are an intervention that addresses school dropout rates among adolescent females or an after-school sports program for the same population. Both of these options may attract greater support in this particular community.

Clarify Objectives

While the overall aim of an intervention remains the same, intervention objectives must flow directly from the specific activities or intervention that will be implemented. In the case of the intervention that seeks to reduce adolescent pregnancy, for instance, whether contraceptive access, a school retention program, or an after-school sports program is selected, the objectives should both reflect what the intervention is and provide a quantitative measure of its impact. Any particular intervention may have several objectives, and they will be specific to the direction that has been selected.

The best goals are written as simple and concise sentences that state what the intervention expects to accomplish (Centers for Disease Control and Prevention [CDC], n.d.). Concrete objectives outline the results that will be reached and the way they will be accomplished. Effective objectives also answer the following questions:

- Who is involved? (usually stated as the population)

- How much change will be accomplished? (usually stated as a percentage)

- What specifically will be accomplished?

- Over what time period will the objective be met? (usually stated as a timeframe). (CDC, n.d.)

A formula for writing specific, measurable, attainable, realistic (or relevant), and time bound (SMART) objectives is: By *[time frame]*, *[a specific target population]* will *[accomplish an outcome based on the intervention goal]*, as evidenced by *[measurable outcome: number, rate, or percentage of change].* For more information on writing **SMART objectives,** see www.cdc.gov/dhdsp/state_program/evaluation_guides/smart_objectives.htm.

If the intervention seeks to decrease adolescent pregnancy by increasing high school graduation rates, specific objectives might read as follows:

- After participating in 80 percent of the after-school academic support activities, 70 percent of the participating students will show a positive change in attitude toward graduating from high school (measured by pre-post survey).

- Increase interest in health careers among fifty at-risk adolescent girls by implementing a speaker's program of graduates who have been successful by the year 20XX.

- By March 15, 20XX, conduct two field trips to local academic institutions or training academies for at least fifty at-risk adolescent girls in Middletown High School.

If the intervention seeks to decrease pregnancy risk by improving access to contraceptives, specific objectives might read as follows:

- By end of academic year 20XX, increase condom availability to students at Middletown High School by providing condoms at three student-attended events (one in school and two out of school).

- By 20XX, the school-based health center will increase from two to four the number of contraceptive methods offered to Middletown High School students.

- By 20XX, conduct two one-day workshops on improving communication skills about sexuality issues for at least 90 percent of parents of students at Middletown High School.

If the intervention content is based on a program identified in the literature to increase participation in organized sports, specific objectives might read as follows:

- During the 20XX academic year, launch a fall or spring semester (or yearlong) all-girl sports program with an initial target population of fifty girls from Middletown High School.

- By 20XX, arrange for a female sports figure to provide both a motivational session to an all-girl assembly session and five small-group discussion and action sessions at Middletown High School.

We hope these examples clarify the importance of preparatory research. While overall goals describe an intervention's general purpose, objectives describe the specific changes that will be implemented as a result of the intervention. Use of previous research supports and informs the intervention.

Determine the Fit of an Existing Intervention

After reviewing the literature, practitioners must decide whether an intervention can meet the needs of the target population. Since there is tremendous variety among communities, some degree of change must generally be made to tailor or adapt an intervention to a target area. A goal in adapting or tailoring an existing intervention is to maintain as high a degree of **fidelity** to the original design, content, and implementation plan as possible to increase the chances of success and effectiveness. A common reason for modification is the length of the original intervention. A two-hour program, for instance, is probably too long if the time available for the current community intervention occurs after weekly prenatal clinic sessions. Likewise, a ten-week intervention that builds on weekly information and interactions may not be appropriate for a detention facility that has considerable weekly turnover.

The appropriateness of the intervention content to a specific racial or ethnic group should also be considered. A faith-based physical activity intervention for African American women would not be inherently appropriate for use with new immigrants from refugee camps in the Middle East, because of cultural differences. Other factors such as age- and gender-appropriateness can also affect the way participants experience interventions. The content of a dating violence intervention aimed at adolescent girls would vary greatly from one aimed at boys. Similarly, since early adolescents are at very different developmental stages from late adolescents, an intervention for sixteen- to eighteen-year-olds would benefit from a different presentation method from one for eleven- to thirteen-year-olds.

Another aspect to consider is needed resources. If highly trained facilitators are essential for intervention effectiveness, the proposed intervention must have the financial resources to pay for this resource. If indoor space is necessary for a physical activity intervention, access to an appropriate venue must be arranged in advance.

Because it is challenging to replicate an intervention in its entirety, several strategies are recommended to help minimize the risk of reducing intervention effectiveness while still maintaining fidelity to the original content (O'Connor, Small, & Cooney, 2007). The best and most obvious approach is to select an intervention that requires little or no modification. Review the adopted intervention components, including the guiding framework, intervention materials, duration, and delivery tactics, to see whether these are congruent with the community and the needs that are being addressed. Involve the staff members who will be responsible for carrying out intervention implementation, as their work can directly affect intervention fidelity. If possible, get guidance from the practitioner who implemented the original intervention. This person can offer insights on where changes can be made that will not alter the intervention's integrity (O'Connor et al., 2007).

A LOGIC MODEL AS AN ORGANIZING STRATEGY

After an intervention approach has been selected, it is helpful to lay out the key features of the intervention using a program planning tool called a **logic model,** which provides a graphic depiction of the rationale behind an intervention. Logic models have been used by intervention planners and evaluators to measure performance and communicate intervention components to staff, stakeholders, and potential funders (Kaplan & Garrett, 2005).

As a planning tool, logic models offer many benefits. For instance, the process of developing a logic model provides the practitioner with a clear understanding of the intervention's purpose, importance, necessary implementation steps, and intended results (W. K. Kellogg Foundation, 2004). As a model is developed, gaps in the intervention plan are easily identified, and a focus on the outcomes is maintained. Since logic models show the outcomes that are expected from each segment of the intervention, the model can also be used to develop an evaluation plan (Taylor-Powell, Jones, & Henert, 2002). A logic model helps create a common understanding of the intervention for all those involved by providing a common language of concepts and terminology that facilitates communication and cohesion during implementation activities. The model serves as a reminder of the interconnections between the various components of an intervention.

There are three distinct approaches to constructing a logic model, with some approaches more appropriate for different stages of an intervention (W. K. Kellogg Foundation, 2004).

- **Theory approach models** use theory to guide the planning and design of an intervention. These models provide a rationale for the programmatic approaches being pursued and set out the intervention strategy that includes what is to be done, how it is to be done, who will carry out the activities, and when the activities will be carried out. These models also explain how and why interventions have been effective in the past. The theory approach to models is frequently used for planning and designing new interventions (W. K. Kellogg Foundation, 2004).

- **Outcome approach models** focus on intended outcomes, which are distinguished in terms of time—from immediate to midterm and long-term outcomes. They illustrate how intervention components will be evaluated to determine if they are achieving their intended results. These models are commonly used for evaluation purposes (W. K. Kellogg Foundation, 2004).

- **Activities approach models** focus on the activities of the project and the expected results from these activities, as well as the resources that are needed for intervention operations. This approach is often used for intervention management (W. K. Kellogg Foundation, 2004).

Components of a Logic Model

While there are different approaches to the construction of a logic model, most will contain the following components: assumptions, situation, inputs, activities, reach, outputs, and outcomes. These components are shown in Table 8.1.

Organizational Strategies for Logic Models

When designing a logic model the aim is to organize the components so that their connections are visible and manageable (Taylor-Powell, 1999). For example, logic models

TABLE 8.1   **Components of a logic model**

Assumptions	Based on beliefs about a program that need to be explicated and coordinated with the program's anticipated goals.
Situation	Explains the purpose of the program; identifies the problem that is to be addressed, also known as the problem statement; articulates not only the various aspects of the problem—such as who is being affected, where the problem is occurring, and when it is occurring—but also how the problem can be solved.
Inputs lead to outputs	Resources, contributions, and investments needed to carry out programmatic activities; common inputs include human resources (such as staff, volunteers, and faculty), fiscal resources (such as public or private monies and donations), material resources (such as space, computer equipment, and other equipment), intellectual property (such as preexisting training modules, curricula, and research results), and involved partners or collaborators (such as health agencies, community organizations, and academic institutions).
Outputs include both activities and reach	**Activities** describe what the program will do and who will benefit, including products, programs, and services that will be employed, such as trainings that will take place, curricula that will be developed, and partnerships that will be forged. **Reach** describes the target population that will receive or participate in the program activities.
Outcomes	Results of the program; can be short term (emerge one to three years after implementation, such as change in knowledge and development of skills), intermediate term (occur four to six years after implementation, such as policies adopted and changes in organizational structure), and long term (emerge after seven to ten years of implementation, such as improved economic, social, and environmental conditions).

Sources: Friis & Sellers, 2004; W. K. Kellogg Foundation, 2004; McCawley, n.d.

can be designed using tables with columns that read from left to right. This format allows planners to visually identify how model components influence each other. Lines and arrows can be used to emphasis special connections between components. Numbered lists might also be employed to draw attention to sequences, such as tasks that need to be specified within a particular component. Using shapes such as circles, ellipses, and boxes to visualize different model components can also be helpful. Tables 8.2, 8.3, 8.4, and 8.5 illustrate four logic models that use tables with columns and lines (Taylor-Powell, 1999).

A FICTIONAL COMMUNITY ASSESSMENT: ADOLESCENT TOBACCO USE

To demonstrate how a logic model's components function, the following hypothetical situation will identify and explain how each component comes into play as an intervention is being designed. As outlined here, the community assessment informs which health problem will be addressed.

A community assessment was recently conducted with Community X in State Y, and data revealed that compared to the rest of the state, Community X had higher overall rates of tobacco use among its adolescents. At the same time, the assessment revealed considerable evidence of low compliance with laws prohibiting tobacco sales to minors among Community X retailers. In light of this information, the Sunshine Organization, a youth-focused community-based organization, in conjunction with Community X Middle School, proposed the Y-Start Now Program, a community-based intervention.

Inputs for the Y-Start Now Program

A variety of community *inputs* could be leveraged to address the problem of tobacco among adolescents in Community X. For instance:

Inputs provided by Community X Middle School include an established School Wellness Council:

▪ In 2005 Community X Middle School established a School Wellness Council in response to the 2005 legislative mandate (the Child Nutrition and WIC Reauthorization Act), which required all schools that participate in school meal programs to establish a childhood obesity school wellness policy. While the council developed a childhood obesity policy, it did not address tobacco prevention due to lack of resources. To fill this gap in resources, the council has partnered with a community-based organization called the Sunshine Organization.

Inputs provided by the Sunshine Organization include staff and volunteers:

▪ Sunshine staff involved in the proposed intervention will oversee the planning, implementation, and evaluation of the intervention. These individuals will also administer school staff trainings. Sunshine's health staff, which has expertise in adolescent health issues, will identify, adapt, and develop intervention educational resources and other related materials in collaboration with Wellness Council members. In addition, Sunshine Youth volunteers will work in coordination with Sunshine staff to assist with intervention-related activities. Both the Sunshine organization and the Community X Middle School will provide space for group meetings.

The Situation

The Y-Start Now planners conduct a literature review and gain knowledge of the health problem as follows:

- In the United States, smoking is the leading cause of preventable illness, disability, and death (CDC, 2009).

- Each day approximately four thousand youth aged twelve to seventeen initiate cigarette smoking (Blank, 2007).

- A broad consensus holds that adolescence is a critical time for tobacco prevention, since almost 70 percent of smokers first try cigarettes during their teens (CDC, 1994b; Spoth, Randall, Trudeau, Shin, & Redmond, 2008).

- To prevent initiation of tobacco use among young people, multilevel strategies are required, particularly interventions that integrate tobacco prevention education, efforts to decrease tobacco sales to minors, and tobacco-free school policies (Nilsson, Stenlund, Bergström, Weinehall, & Janlert, 2006).

- Considering that adolescents spend a significant portion of their day in the classroom, schools are an ideal setting to implement an intervention that will help them avoid tobacco use (CDC, 1994a).

- Increasing retail store owners' compliance with youth tobacco access laws will decrease adolescents' ability to purchase tobacco products. Such compliance can help delay or prevent adolescent tobacco use (Jason, Ji, Anes, & Birkhead, 1991).

Example Logic Models for Four Ecological Domains

The Y-Start Now program will intervene at different ecological levels of influence, including the group, organization, community, and policy levels (see Chapter Four). The overall intervention goal will be to prevent or delay the initiation of smoking among middle school children living in Community X. Each logic model will describe the ecological domain's inputs, objectives, activities, reach, outputs, and outcomes, as well as the intervention goal, objective(s), situation, and assumptions.

The first ecological domain of the proposed intervention will focus on the group level. According to the literature, increased knowledge of the consequences of tobacco use has an impact on students' attitudes to and beliefs about cigarette use and equips adolescents with skills to reject social pressures. Such education decreases the risk that young people will initiate tobacco use (Luepker, Johnson, Murray, & Pechacek, 1983). The group-level objective seeks a 70 percent increase, within one year, in pre-posttest awareness of tobacco consequences and skills to avoid tobacco initiation among students in Community X Middle School.

- Inputs and resources related to this domain include existing curricula regarding tobacco prevention among adolescents; Community X Middle School health education staff; Sunshine's health staff, who have expertise in adolescent health issues; and the existing partnership between Community X Middle School and the Sunshine Organization.

- Activities to achieve these objectives include creating a tobacco prevention education curriculum tailored to the needs of Community X Middle School students (the target group); conducting tobacco prevention education at Community X Middle School as part of the daily health education curriculum. These activities will reach middle school students.

- Outputs or results flow from a combination of activities and reach.

- The expected outcomes are an increase in knowledge, awareness, and assertiveness skills, as well as a decrease in the initiation of cigarette smoking among Community X Middle School students.

Table 8.2 shows the layout of the logic model for the **group-level domain** of the proposed intervention.

The second ecological domain of the proposed intervention will focus on the organizational level. According to the literature, schools that require that their general health education courses include tobacco education are more effective in discouraging smoking among middle school students (Walter, Vaugh, & Wynder, 1989). The organization-level objective of the proposed intervention is that by 20XX, all health education courses offered at Community X Middle School will offer tobacco prevention education.

- Inputs and resources related to this domain include existing train-the-trainer curricula on tobacco prevention education and Community X Middle School health education staff.

- Activities to achieve this objective include adapting a train-the-trainer program that equips Community X health education teachers with the tools to conduct tobacco prevention education; training trainers to provide tobacco prevention education in middle school health education classes. These activities will reach health education staff.

TABLE 8.2 Logic Model: Group-level domain

Program goal	To prevent or delay the initiation of smoking among middle school children living in Community X.
Group-level objective	By year 20XX, a 70 percent increase in pre-posttest awareness of tobacco consequences and skills to avoid tobacco initiation among students in Community X Middle School.

	Inputs	Outputs		Outcomes
	Invested resources ⟶	Activities ⟶ undertaken	Reach	
	Existing tobacco prevention curricula	Tailor existing tobacco prevention education curriculum	Middle school pupils	
	Community X Middle School health staff	Provide tobacco prevention education to middle school students as part of health education sessions		
	Sunshine health staff's expertise in youth health education			
	Existing partnership between Community X Middle School and Sunshine Organization			

Situation — Compared to the rest of the state, Community X has higher overall rates of cigarette use among adolescents.

Evaluation — Process ↔ Impact ↔ Outcome

Assumption: After middle school students receive information about tobacco consequences and skill-building training on peer pressure avoidance, they will be better prepared to delay cigarette initiation.

Source: Adapted from Taylor-Powell, 1999.

■ Outputs are reflected by a combination of activities and reach.

■ The expected outcomes are an increase in knowledge and competency skills among middle school health education teachers.

Table 8.3 shows the layout of the logic model for the **organization-level domain** of the proposed intervention.

The third ecological level of the proposed intervention will focus on the community level. Study reports have confirmed that local community retail cigarette vendors were more compliant with local ordinances to restrict tobacco sales to minors when the vendors were provided with information about youth access laws (Keay, Woodruff, Wildey, & Kenney, 1993; Stead & Lancaster, 2000; Wildey et al., 1995; Woodruff, Erickson, Wildey, & Kenney, 1993). Likewise, other studies note that reducing minors' community access to cigarettes can decrease smoking among adolescent smokers (CDC, 1994b; DiFranza, 1992; Jason et al., 1991; Stanton, Mahalski, McGee, & Silva, 1993). The first community-level objective is to increase, within six months of intervention initiation, vendor awareness of laws prohibiting sales of tobacco to minors. The second community-level objective is to reduce, within one year of intervention initiation, cigarette sales to minors by 30 percent in stores that received the intervention.

■ The inputs and resources related to this domain include existing education and training curricula—in particular, project TRUST, an evaluated intervention that combines face-to-face trainings and educational materials (Keay et al., 1993; Wildey et al., 1995; Woodruff et al., 1993) regarding tobacco prevention among adolescents—and Sunshine youth volunteers to assist with vendor education and training.

■ The activities to achieve the intervention objectives include adaptation of project TRUST education and training materials to fit the needs of Community X's vendors; recruitment of retail stores who agree to receive three educational sessions; training of Sunshine youth volunteers on project TRUST procedures and materials; and presentation of education and training sessions on youth access laws to local tobacco vendors.

■ These activities will reach merchants who sell tobacco products. In addition, minors who attempt to purchase cigarettes will be targeted.

■ Activities and reach combined reflect outputs.

■ Expected outcomes include an increased compliance with youth access laws among vendors who participate in the Y-Start Now program. The intervention will also decrease cigarette access to minors who attempt to purchase cigarettes at retail stores that participate in the proposed intervention.

Table 8.4 shows the layout of the logic model for the **community-level domain** of the proposed intervention.

TABLE 8.3   **Logic Model: Organization-level domain**

Program goal	To prevent or delay the initiation of smoking among middle school children living in Community X.
Organization-level objectives	By 2011, all health education courses offered at Community X Middle School will offer tobacco prevention education.

		Inputs	Outputs		Outcomes
Situation	Compared to the rest of the state, Community X has higher overall rates of cigarette use among adolescents.	Invested resources ⟶	Activities ⟶ undertaken	Reach	Evaluation Process ←→ Impact ←→ Outcome
		Existing train-the-trainer middle school tobacco prevention curricula	Tailor existing tobacco prevention education curriculum	Health education staff	
		Community X Middle School health staff	Train middle school health education trainers		
			Conduct tobacco prevention education in middle school health education classes		

Assumption: Middle school teachers who participate in trainer workshops will incorporate tobacco prevention education in their education classes.

Source: Adapted from Taylor-Powell, 1999.

TABLE 8.4 Logic Model Community-level domain

Program goal	To prevent or delay the initiation of smoking among middle school children living in Community X.		
Community-level objectives	1. Increase, within six months of intervention initiation, vendor awareness of laws prohibiting sales of tobacco to minors. 2. Reduce, within one year of program initiation, cigarette sales to minors in Community X by 30 percent in stores that received the intervention.		

Situation	Inputs	Outputs		Outcomes
Compared to the rest of the state, Community X has higher overall rates of cigarette use among adolescents.	Invested resources →	Activities undertaken →	Reach	Evaluation Process ↔ Impact ↔ Outcome
	Existing education and training curricula	Tailor existing education and training materials	Local merchants	
	Sunshine youth volunteers	Recruit retail stores that agree to receive three educational sessions Train Sunshine youth volunteers to conduct outreach		
	Sunshine staff	Conduct education and training sessions on youth access laws to local tobacco vendors		

Assumption 1: When provided with information about youth access laws, vendors will be more compliant with local ordinances to restrict tobacco sales to minors.

Assumption 2: Reducing minors' community access to cigarettes will reduce smoking among adolescents.

Source: Adapted from Taylor-Powell, 1999.

The fourth ecological level of this proposed intervention focuses on the policy level. Current research findings regarding tobacco-free school policies show that students who attend schools with tobacco-free school policies are less likely to use tobacco than students in schools without a tobacco-free school policy (Pentz et al., 1989; Wakefield et al., 2000). The policy-level objective notes that by 2012, Community X Middle School will adopt a tobacco-free school policy that will prohibit tobacco use on and around school property.

- The inputs and resources related to this domain include the existence of the School Wellness Council at Community X Middle School and their past experience with developing and implementing a childhood obesity policy; the existing partnership between Sunshine Organization and the School Wellness Council, whose designated leaders include the school principal, the health education teachers, and the PTA chair; and the existence of school policy toolkits.

- The activities to achieve intervention objectives include obtaining necessary buy-ins and approvals for the tobacco-free school policy from key members of the school community; collaborating with the School Wellness Council to create a tobacco-free school policy; collaborating with the School Wellness Council to create an implementation plan for the tobacco-free school policy; and implementing the tobacco-free school policy.

- These activities will reach both the staff and students at Community X Middle School.

- Activities and reach combined reflect outputs.

- Expected outcomes include decreased rates of cigarette smoking initiation in the student population at Community X Middle School.

Table 8.5 shows the layout of the logic model for the **policy-level domain** of the proposed interventions.

SUMMARY

This chapter covered the issues that practitioners must take into account before adopting and implementing an intervention to address a target population's health issue(s). It highlighted the importance of conducting adequate research, as well as considering the appropriateness of existing interventions. Once an approach is selected, a logic model offers an opportunity to develop a plan based on clearly defined intervention goals and SMART objectives.

TABLE 8.5   **Logic Model: Policy-level domain**

Program goal	To prevent or delay the initiation of smoking among middle school children living in Community X.
Policy-level objectives	By 2012, Community X Middle School will adopt a tobacco-free school policy that will prohibit tobacco use on and around school property.

		Inputs	Outputs		Outcomes	
		Invested resources →	Activities undertaken ——→	Reach		
Situation	Compared to the rest of the state, Community X has higher overall rates of cigarette use among adolescents.	Existence of school policy toolkits	Outreach efforts to gain buy-in from key members of the school community	Both the staff and students at Community X Middle School	Process ↔ Impact ↔ Outcome	Evaluation
		Existing School Wellness Council at Community X Middle School, which in the past developed and implemented a childhood obesity policy	Create a tobacco-free school policy Create an implementation plan for the created tobacco-free policy			
		Existing partnership between Sunshine Organization and School Wellness Council members	Implement the tobacco-free policy			

Assumption: Students who attend schools with tobacco-free school policies are less likely to use tobacco.

Source: Adapted from Taylor-Powell, 1999.

KEY TERMS

Activities

Activities approach models

Assumptions

Boolean operators

CINAHL

Cochrane Review

Community Guide

Community-level domain

EMBASE

Fidelity

Global Health

Google Scholar

Group-level domain

Inputs

Logic model

National Guideline Clearinghouse

Networking

Organization-level domain

Outcome approach models

Outputs include both activities and reach

Overall goal

Policy-level domain

Problem statement

Public Health Partners

PubMed

Reach

Scientific literature

SMART objectives

Theory approach models

Web of Science

ACTIVITIES

1. Explain what is wrong with the following objectives:

    a. Help cancer patients feel better when they lose their hair.

    b. Decrease deaths due to cardiovascular disease.

2. How would you rewrite the preceding objectives into SMART objectives?

3. Develop a logic model for a community-based health intervention. First identify intervention goals (for example, to decrease diabetes). Then identify two SMART program objectives (such as increasing fruit and vegetable consumption and increasing regular exercise). Develop at least three activities for each objective (such as offering free cooking lessons). Specify how intervention activities will meet intervention objectives and how the objectives will meet the intervention goals.

DISCUSSION QUESTIONS

1. Discuss the issues you need to consider when adopting an existing intervention to avoid implementing an intervention that is inappropriate for your target population.

2. Drawing from the hypothetical Y-Start Now intervention discussed in this chapter, imagine you are a high school principal in Community X and you are interested in

launching an intervention that aims to prevent or delay the initiation of smoking among high school kids living in your community. Review the Y-Start Now sample logic model for four ecological domains and discuss the following questions:

a. What individual(s), group(s), and organization(s) would you partner with, if any?

b. What components of the existing Y-Start Now intervention would you keep or build upon? Which components would you change, and why?

c. Describe new approaches and activities that you would employ.

CHAPTER

9

IMPLEMENTING A COMMUNITY-BASED INTERVENTION

LEARNING OBJECTIVES

- Become familiar with the steps necessary to implement a community intervention at four different ecological levels
- Understand different strategies appropriate for recruiting intervention participants
- Identify three different community venues in which to carry out a health intervention

OVERVIEW

This chapter will cover the steps necessary to implement a community-based intervention in each of the four ecological focus areas. Strategies to avoid or overcome common problems will be discussed as the intervention moves from inception to implementation.

IMPLEMENTATION AT THE FOUR ECOLOGICAL LEVELS

Interventions to address community-based health problems can be implemented at any of the four ecological levels—group, institution, community, or policy (see Chapter Four). In reviewing the literature, it is clear that a variety of strategies and interventions can be implemented at each level to address almost every conceivable health problem with which a community might be faced. After choosing the ecological level and the specific intervention of interest, it is finally time to start the implementation activities. Table 9.1 presents examples of possible interventions to address the community health problem of high rates of obesity at each ecological level that will be used as an example for implementation strategies.

It is important to develop a plan to organize all the activities that will be involved in implementing an intervention. The steps necessary to implement an intervention at the group and organization levels are similar to each other and distinct from the steps necessary at the community or policy level.

TABLE 9.1   **Interventions to decrease obesity at four ecological levels**

Ecological Focus Area	Proposed Intervention
Group	Arrange a four-session dance class among immigrants who attend a local community center
Organization	Organize a committee at a local school whose goal is to increase physical activity among students and staff
Community	Build a community walking path
Policy	List calorie counts and heart-healthy choices on all restaurant menus

Interventions at the Group or Organization Level

For group- and institution-level interventions, it is important to develop a plan that will ensure that materials, trained staff, and other resources are available before beginning to field the intervention. Developing a **timeline** for the entire project and a **recruitment plan** for identifying participants should ideally be done before the start of intervention activities.

A **Gantt chart,** which is a type of timeline, details in visual form the anticipated start and stop dates for intervention activities. A sample timeline for an intervention funded for one year using dance as physical activity with immigrant women is presented in Table 9.2.

TABLE 9.2   **One-year implementation timeline**

Activity	1	2	3	4	5	6	7	8	9	10	11	12
Obtain IRB approval	×	×										
Hire one half-time staff member	×	×										
Develop recruitment plan	×											
Finalize arrangements for intervention venue, supplies, and equipment	×											
Copy pre-post evaluation instruments and educational materials	×											
Recruit participants		×	×	×	×	×	×	×	×	×		
Offer intervention activities			×	×	×	×	×	×	×	×	×	
Input data				×	×	×	×	×	×	×	×	
Conduct preliminary data analysis							×					
Conduct final data analysis											×	
Write final report											×	×
Disseminate findings												×

While it may seem that activities such as obtaining institutional review board approval and hiring staff are fairly straightforward, it is *very* important to acknowledge that everything is likely to take longer than expected. It is better to be realistic and, if things go more smoothly than expected, have an additional creative activity developed to fill the extra time, than it is to be way behind in month three of a one-year intervention.

The following six implementation steps are suggested for community health interventions. For the example in Table 9.2, steps shown are in the ecological focus areas of groups or organizations.

Content, Timing, and Logistics

1. *Specify the content, timing, and logistics* of an intervention so that the same material is covered in the same way each time the intervention is offered. If the intervention is offering dance classes to a group of new immigrants, decide on the best approach to engage the target population in the intervention. In terms of timing of content, for example, would it be better to have music going as people come into the room, to get them into an appropriate mind-set? Or would it be better to begin with formal introductions and a discussion of the project, and then begin music? Discuss with collaborators the length and timing of the presentation. Logistics would include reserving the community center for the appropriate times and order and have available any videos and educational brochures in the appropriate language(s). Try the videos out on an office machine or, better still, on the machine at the intervention site to make certain that it is in working order. Table 9.3 shows a suggested schedule for a dance class whose goal is to increase physical activity among immigrant women.

Think carefully about the content of interventions or curricula used in other settings and how they will have to be adapted for a particular target population. For example, are the ages of people who volunteered as participants homogeneous? Do changes need to be made in the intervention because the population is of a different racial or ethnic group than that of the original intervention? Is the length of a session appropriate for the attention span of participants? Should activities be more varied? How can interaction be maximized? The answers to these questions come from thinking through every activity in the intervention and also knowing the target population well.

Staff Training

2. *Train project staff* who will be implementing the intervention so that they understand the philosophy of the intervention, follow a similar logistics plan, and present identical material and activities to participants. If multiple group leaders are involved, the training session will ensure that those implementing the curriculum have the same understanding about the intervention. Training topics should include the following:

- Protection of human subjects and guidelines of the institutional review board

- The background of the specific health issue that the intervention is attempting to address

- The content of the curriculum developed for the intervention

- The need for uniform implementation of all aspects of the intervention

- The time allocated to each activity and session of the intervention

- How the evaluation data will be collected and managed

A staff training session for a dance class at the group level can be organized like the one shown in Table 9.4.

Participant Recruitment

3. *Develop a recruitment plan* for participants that includes short- and long-term goals. A recruitment plan should include the target number of participants (sample size), ideally based on a power analysis. Web sites are available to do this computation, or you may refer to a standard statistics textbook. If the intervention is occurring over time, oversampling is a good idea to account for **attrition.** A recruitment plan should also detail an initial list of sites where recruitment will occur, what incentives or facilitators, if any, will be available, and the time period in which recruitment is expected to occur. For example, if fifty participants need to be recruited over a one-month period of time, a schedule of the number anticipated each week should be

TABLE 9.3   **Content and schedule for dance class**

Time	Activity	To Do
6:30–7:00	Introductions, individual goals, and administration of pretest	Bring pens, consent forms, and pretests
7:00–7:15	Warm-up exercises	Need stereo and appropriate CDs
7:15–7:20	Break, water	Bring water
7:20–7:45	Dance	
7:45–7:50	Break, water; discuss music choices	
7:45–8:15	Dance	
8:15–8:30	Conclusion Posttest at last session	

developed. While starting slowly is expected, by week two at least twenty participants should be signed up. If this does not go as scheduled, the recruitment plan should be revised, perhaps with additional sites, staff, or incentives.

While health workers may believe that their message will be of intrinsic interest to the target population, it is important to remember that people have many, many competing interests. Health is often not at the top of their agendas because work, chores, children, and family responsibilities will all take priority. Because of these competing concerns, just putting up a sign or handing out flyers will not result in the desired attendance at an intervention session or event.

One recruitment strategy is to identify two or three people from the target population who have an interest in the problem area. If possible, give them some type of leadership role and offer them some small payment for their time. These initial

TABLE 9.4   Staff training schedule

Time	Activity	Things to Bring
8:30–8:45	Welcome and introductions	Name tags
8:45–9:15	Interactive presentation about health issue, obesity, physical activity, and diet	PowerPoint presentation, computer, LCD projector
9:15–9:45	Exercise about cultural competence and the target population	Handouts and props for exercise
9:45–10:00	Break, snack	Beverages, fruit, low-sugar cookies
10:00–11:00	Research ethics	Internet access for group to use instructional module and test
11:00–11:45	Group test for ethics certification	
11:45–12:15	Schedule, recruitment, and data collection	Copies of data forms, calendar
12:15–12:30	Questions and thank-yous	

recruits will play an important role in the recruitment of other participants. If possible, initiate recruitment at an event or site where people of the target population are already gathered for other reasons. Obtaining the cooperation and buy-in of a community leader—especially one who has access to the target population and might personally refer potential participants—is valuable. For example, if immigrant women are the target population, explaining the intervention and working with caseworkers at the resettlement agency and the local community center will facilitate access to this group.

Choose a Venue

Also consider the location where the intervention will be held. A community center is generally a good venue because people are already drawn there for other reasons. The public library should be considered, but is not necessarily a natural gathering place. Consider alternatives such as scheduling the dance class to follow an ESL class or holding the class concurrently with a children's activity so that parents can come early, attend the class, and then pick up their children. Try to schedule recruitment when the target population will be at the intervention site for another reason. Offering an intervention after church services so that people do not have to make a special trip to attend it is an example of this strategy. Also consider scheduling the intervention as part of an elective activity at a local alternative or charter high school.

The use of facilitators and incentives can aid recruitment. Facilitators make it easier for potential participants to attend a program, and they include things like transportation vouchers and child care. Incentives are small perks or gifts that can generate interest in the intervention such as T-shirts, supermarket vouchers, tote bags, or caps with the intervention name. Offering one or two inexpensive raffle prizes purchased from or donated by local merchants or discount stores adds a bit of excitement. Giving away a CD with the music used in the class can also serve as an incentive to practice at home. Providing food certainly makes an intervention more popular and easier for participants to attend.

4. *Line up logistics.* Have a mechanism in place to cover intervention expenses. Check that the venue is available and that supplies are on hand at the time they are needed. Make certain that colleagues or community members who are assisting will be on hand at the appointed time. Even if approval has been obtained from administration, try to tactfully check with the line staff who will be unlocking doors or turning on the heat; miscommunication can occur and is easy to prevent.

The Pilot Study

5. *Conduct a **pilot study,*** a smaller-scale version or practice run of the final intervention, with all the same elements that will be used. The purpose of a pilot study is to test all aspects of the intervention, including the plan for logistics and the evaluation instruments. A pilot study can provide information such as whether the target population will actually show up for an intervention, how participants respond to the

message or material, whether the program is too long or short, and whether the pretest and posttest used for evaluation are understandable and of appropriate length.

An observer who takes extensive notes during the pilot study will provide important feedback on aspects that are not visible to the person actually leading a group. A debriefing session with the intervention team can be scheduled immediately after the pilot study to elicit suggestions for changes and opinions about what did and did not work. If extensive changes are indicated, consider conducting a second pilot study after the changes have been integrated into the intervention, for greater assurances of a smooth flow when the intervention goes into the field.

6. *Develop a data management plan.* Collect at least a minimal amount of data during the pilot study to permit a data management plan to be developed while the intervention is unfolding (see Chapter Six).

During both a pilot study and the actual intervention, good data management necessitates attention to details. Before leaving the office, remember to bring all necessary forms and more pens or pencils than will be needed, as well as clipboards or another type of hard surface on which to write. If interviews are being audiotaped, be sure that the tape recorder is working before leaving the office and extra tapes and batteries are available. Having a second tape recorder on hand is a very good idea. If a survey is being administered, try to assure that each person has some degree of privacy in which to complete it, either in terms of space (by preventing others from seeing their responses) or in terms of time (by giving participants a longer period of time to complete them). At least one member of the study team should be available to answer questions while participants are completing the survey. As the surveys are completed, scan each one for completeness. If this practice does not seem too intrusive, be aware that this is the only opportunity you will have to ask whether a participant meant to skip certain questions.

Final Details

In addition to the data instruments, two other types of forms must be completed. **Consent forms** are necessary for certain types of studies, indicating approval for the intervention from an institutional review board (IRB). IRB approval ensures that the rights of study participants are not violated, and it must be obtained before even pilot data are collected (Chapter Three). While not every type of intervention will require signed consent forms, in those cases where they are needed, they are often cumbersome and many populations do not readily understand them. For such cases, consider adding a short information sheet for potential participants. This should be written at a reading level appropriate for the population, explaining simply and without jargon what the intervention will entail in terms of time and energy, and why pre- and postintervention data collection is needed.

A second form is a **locator form,** used to contact participants at future dates if indicated as part of the intervention or evaluation. While addresses and phone numbers are enough for some populations, the advent of cell phones has made finding people more difficult, because numbers change frequently and there is no cell-phone directory. To forestall this problem, request the phone numbers or other contact information for one or two friends or close relatives who would know how to reach the participant if the phone number changes. Note the date and site where this information is collected.

INTERVENTIONS AT THE COMMUNITY OR POLICY LEVEL

A different set of steps is suggested for community- or policy-level interventions. Although no two communities are identical, a review of the literature to examine how other communities have become engaged in community-based interventions is useful. Sometimes the problem of concern has received enough press coverage to raise community awareness and concern. Alternatively, political leaders in a community may be using an issue to gain political advantage and appeal to the public for support. It is certainly easier to propose an intervention about a problem that is already of concern to the community than it is to introduce a new issue that most people have not previously considered to be a problem. The following steps need to be taken in developing an intervention at the community or policy level.

Research Policy from Various Sources

1. *Do the homework about the specific health policy.* Research what other organizations and communities have done, as, for example, in Table 9.1, where a group set out to create a community walking path. In addition to the academic literature, scan local newspapers and other media sources, search on the Internet—especially the web pages of local organizations—review records of local and regional conferences and meetings, and check organizational newsletters. Identify listservs that focus on the health issue (see Chapter Eight). Also learn what steps are necessary to change or enact a specific regulation or policy in the targeted community. For example, there may be public land available that could easily be used for the community walking trail. Assess the key players advocating for and against the issue, and find out whether anyone in the intervention group knows these individuals well enough to approach them personally.

2. *Specify the goal, change, policy, or law to be changed.* Use the material gathered to specify the exact change that is desired. It is best to have a definite goal in mind before beginning to lobby for the intervention, which might be to establish a physical activity committee in the local school or to get funding for one walking path within the geographic boundaries of the community.

Determining Resources

3. *Identify and work with others who are interested in the same area.* Stakeholder support is critical for all community interventions, whether the change is targeted for the organization, community, or policy level. Continue to broaden the base of support

by identifying additional groups and using a variety of outlets to publicize meetings, such as local papers and radio stations, tenants associations, church bulletins, and notices on supermarket bulletin boards.

Train project staff to speak publicly about the need for the project at various community public meetings. If it is necessary to organize a meeting for the public on the issue, this will entail a number of logistical challenges to draw a reasonably sized audience. It is helpful to offer something in addition to a meeting agenda, like an informational movie or a speaker from another community who has worked successfully on a similar topic. A debate on a topic between knowledgeable well-known speakers can be useful in sparking both community and media interest. All events should be carefully organized and publicized well in advance through the local media, perhaps in the form of a press release. Before every meeting, check the venue to verify that it is ready and that all the equipment such as slide projectors and microphones are in working order.

4. *Maintain detailed records of meetings, contacts, and discussions.* For community- and policy-level interventions, multiple meetings with stakeholders are a critical part of the plan to gain support for a communitywide intervention or policy change. However, it is easy to get caught up in the urgency of responding to deadlines, planning meetings, and instrument development and forget about documenting exactly what transpired. No matter how pressured you are, it is important to maintain records of all meetings, publicity, flyers, and planning notes, so that the group will have a sense of the amount of work done and how far they have come. These records can also form the basis of an evaluation report (see Chapter Ten). If the initial attempts at change are not successful, these records will enable the group to consider new options and continue their efforts by building on the work that has been done.

5. *Present a proposal on the desired change or intervention to the appropriate planning board, legislative body, or government agency.* The background research will have provided guidance on the recommended format for presentation of the proposed changes. Be sure to have several people review the written proposal or oral presentation and allow enough time to integrate their suggestions.

If the plan or proposed change is not accepted, it will be necessary to assess the organizational strategy and revise and repeat steps 4 and 5 in order to address objections that were raised or shortcomings that were identified.

SUMMARY

This chapter has received the steps necessary for practitioners to implement interventions to address community-based health problems at each of the four ecological levels: group, institution, community, and policy. Careful planning is called for as each step is taken to implement the intervention.

KEY TERMS

Attrition
Consent forms
Gantt chart
Locator form

Pilot study
Recruitment plan
Timeline

ACTIVITIES

Oral health is an aspect of immigrant health care that is often overlooked. Lack of access to proper dental care, changing cultural norms regarding eating practices, and the general transition to the United States create challenges. Pick an immigrant population from one U.S. city and complete the following activities:

1. Name one intervention for this population and this health problem that is focused at the group and organization levels. Identify what ingredients—staff, financial and other resources, and time frame—would be necessary to successfully implement the intervention.

2. Interventions on the community and policy levels are often linked. Review city and state health department materials and describe any community planning currently underway for oral health. Identify relevant policies that might influence access to care.

DISCUSSION QUESTIONS

1. Outline a recruitment and retention plan for an intervention to lower the high school dropout rate in a specific community.

2. Discuss three possible reasons why the implementation of a health intervention might fail.

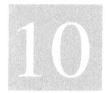

EVALUATING A COMMUNITY-BASED INTERVENTION

LEARNING OBJECTIVES

- Understand the basic components of an evaluation plan
- Distinguish between information gathered for a process evaluation, an impact evaluation, and an outcome evaluation
- Become familiar with the value of triangulated data
- Explain how to disseminate results of an evaluation

OVERVIEW

This chapter will discuss why an evaluation is an essential part of any community-based intervention. Information will be provided about the methods and formats in which to frame an evaluation.

REASONS FOR EVALUATION

Evaluation is a necessary component of a community-based health intervention when the hope is to develop it into a sustainable intervention. An evaluation is a systematic assessment of the effectiveness of an intervention or policy.

Evaluations can be developed either to assess or to find areas of improvement for an intervention that has been implemented. Evaluations can also assess the benefits of an intervention in relation to the costs and resources allocated. If a pilot project has been developed to secure funding for a larger effort, evaluators can provide evidence demonstrating that objectives have been or can be achieved. Positive evaluation findings are likely to convince funders that their money was well spent, and such findings might encourage their further support for the project because they validate their investment. In addition, proving to various stakeholders such as community leaders and politicians that the intervention achieved its goals is the best way to argue for continued and even permanent funding.

Types of Evaluation

There are three types of evaluation design. A **process evaluation** is designed to inform the practitioner how the intervention is going, indicating which aspects are working as planned and which might need to be revised to reach the project's objectives. An **impact evaluation** examines whether the short-term objectives have been achieved. To attribute causality to the intervention, an impact evaluation calls for a comparison with a similar population that has not been exposed to the intervention, and this evaluation is carried out at the same time as the intervention. Data collected during an impact evaluation allow for feedback to improve the intervention while it is underway and guide the practitioner toward modification of the intervention if the objectives are not being met. The third type of evaluation, an **outcome evaluation,** is conducted at the end of the project to determine whether the overall objectives have been achieved. It should answer the question of whether the outcomes can be attributed to the intervention rather than to other factors occurring around the same time. The results of an outcome evaluation will also determine if there are any unintended outcomes, either positive or negative, from the intervention. An outcome evaluation should be able to assess the costs versus the benefits of the intervention after the intervention has been completed.

The different types of interventions ask distinct questions. If, for example, the intervention is a retraining program for people who have lost their jobs and have been out of work for over a year, a process evaluation would ask the following questions:

1. What is the content of the training?

2. How are the trainees being selected?

3. How is the training being conducted?

4. Are the roles of the project staff clearly defined?

5. What materials and procedures are being used by the trainers, and are they being used in the same way by all the trainers?

6. What are the intervention staff's perceptions of how the training is going, and how do they think it might be improved?

7. Are the training sessions well attended?

An impact evaluation, on the other hand, would assess the following:

1. How much of the information is being retained by the client?

2. Has the client learned new skills?

3. Do the clients seem more positive about being able to find a job after they have acquired the new skills?

4. Has the client actually used the newly acquired skills to look for a job?

Finally, an outcome evaluation might be undertaken after a substantial period of time has elapsed since the clients have completed the job training intervention to determine the following:

1. The proportion of the clients actually in the workforce

2. The length of time that the clients have been able to hold onto the job after being hired

3. The reasons that some of the clients have not been able to hold onto a job since completing the training

Potential Evaluators

An evaluation can be provided by the intervention team or by an outside team of people hired to perform the evaluation. The evaluation is more convincing to the public when neutral outsiders who are less likely than project staff to have a personal interest in the project's success collect and analyze the data for the evaluation. However, if the researchers need the data to track the progress of the intervention and give frequent feedback to the practitioners rather than convince others to support the intervention, using project staff as evaluators is appropriate and usually less costly. Conducting an evaluation means that designing an evaluation plan, developing or identifying instruments that can be used for the evaluation, collecting the data, and performing the data analysis must all be performed in addition to the work of implementing the intervention.

Regardless of how and by whom the results of the intervention will be used, the evaluation plan should be developed concurrent to the intervention. Making the evaluation an integral part of the overall intervention will avoid a common pitfall of lacking **baseline data** for comparison. It will allow feedback of information during the course of the implementation and encourage all team members to become familiar with the evaluation goals. In addition, thinking about evaluation at the same time that the intervention is being designed allows any evaluation expenses that will be incurred to be included in the proposed budget. Most funding agencies today require some kind of accountability of their funded projects and allow researchers to spend 5 to 10 percent of the overall budget on evaluation items.

PREPARING FOR AN EVALUATION

It is important to involve the advisory group and other stakeholders in the evaluation discussion and design as soon as planning the evaluation starts. This may take some time and effort because people who have never been engaged in research may not be acquainted with the rules of scientific objectivity. The rules of data collection and how an evaluation will increase the credibility of the outcomes will require some explanation to these groups. Some basic concepts of the research design and the importance of protection of human subjects will also require discussion. All this groundwork will increase the likelihood that the stakeholders will support an evaluation of the intervention.

The research team must develop an evaluation plan with a budget and timeline to enable the process to move forward in a systematic manner. Examples of two timelines for one-year interventions at the institution and the policy level appear in the next section.

DESIGNING THE EVALUATION

Four steps are required in developing an evaluation design. Each of these is described in turn in this section.

Step 1: Setting a Timeline

A **Gantt chart** is a type of timeline that details the anticipated start and stop dates for evaluation in visual form. It can be shown in units of weeks, months, or years. A sample timeline for an evaluation of a one-year intervention using dance classes as a form of exercise in a senior center to increase stamina and mobility appears in Table 10.1.

Step 2: Establishing Which Objectives and Outcomes to Evaluate

As a next step, list objectives and specific aims or outcomes of the intervention that will be evaluated. The goal of an intervention pertains to the problem that will be addressed, such as decreasing adolescent pregnancies, reducing cigarette smoking, or

TABLE 10.1   **Sample evaluation timeline**

Activity	Month												
	Jan	Feb	Mar	Apr	May	June	July	Aug	Sept	Oct	Nov	Dec	1 Year Later
Process Evaluation Activities													
Hire or train staff members to conduct evaluation	X												
Determine whether required number of dance instructors has been hired and trained		X	X										
Determine whether the required number of dance classes was held (review class roster)					X	X	X	X	X	X	X		
Analyze the data and feedback for practitioners							X	X	X	X	X	X	
Impact Evaluation Activities													
Develop instrument to determine whether change occurred				X	X	X							
Collect and analyze data					X	X	X	X	X	X	X		
Outcome Evaluation Activities													
Develop instrument and determine whether change has been sustained													X

improving cardiovascular health. The objectives refer to the strategies that will be used to address the problem, such as increasing opportunities for after-school activities for girls (to address the problem or overall aim of reducing adolescent pregnancy), implementing tobacco-cessation interventions in community libraries (to address the problem or overall aim of reducing cigarette smoking), or organizing a church-based walking intervention for women (to address the problem of women's declining cardiovascular health). Recall from Chapter Eight that specific goals can vary depending on the ecological focus of the intervention (whether at the group, institution, community, or policy level). In reviewing the specific objectives of the intervention, consider the results of the community assessment (Chapter Seven), feasibility of the intervention, access to the target population, and available resources. All these aspects should be considered when you are deciding which aspect of the intervention to evaluate.

Step 3: Determining the Appropriate Type of Evaluation

A process evaluation assesses the progress of the project and how well the intervention is being implemented. Process data can be collected from recruitment logs, participant records, the minutes of project staff meetings, and individual or group interviews with staff members, stakeholders, and members of the target population. Observational techniques can provide information about how the activities are being implemented and the degree of **fidelity** to the intervention protocol and design.

An impact evaluation investigates whether the intervention achieved its objectives. This type of evaluation requires careful selection of the data to be collected and the indicators to be used for data analysis. It is likely that **quantitative methods** will be used for this type of evaluation, which necessitates identifying instruments such as questionnaires that will measure the relevant constructs. Once collected, responses can be easily downloaded into a data software program (such as Stata, SPSS, or SAS) and analyzed for **statistical significance**.

Qualitative methods can be used for impact evaluation. These include strategies such as participant observation, focus groups, and **semistructured interviews**, in which text data are analyzed for recurrent themes. **Triangulation of methods—** using both quantitative and qualitative methods to examine different facets of the intervention—is also possible. The type of methodology selected depends on what is being measured and the resources and time available for measurement.

The strongest quantitative method for evaluating whether an intervention has achieved its goals is a **randomized-controlled trial.** It is considered the gold standard for experimental research because it is the least likely to produce biased results. However, few community-based interventions can use this method because of the amount of resources needed. In a randomized-controlled trial, both an experimental unit and a control unit of analysis must be identified and randomly assigned. The **experimental group** receives the intervention, and the **control group** is either left alone (except for data collection) or given some kind of **placebo** treatment, which should have no effect. This design is expensive because it involves twice as many subjects or organizations, depending on the unit of analysis, so that the two groups can be compared to determine whether the intervention had an effect. Most of the cost of this research design depends on the required sample size, the **unit of analysis,** and the efforts necessary for follow-up.

Quasi-experimental designs are more realistic but still strong quantitative methods for evaluating community interventions (Shadish, Cook, & Campbell, 2002). The strongest form of quasi-experimental design is one in which the evaluator selects a comparison group that is similar in many respects to the intervention group. No randomization is involved, and baseline data are collected from both groups prior to the start of any intervention activities. This is called a **two-group/pre-post design.** A one-group/**pre-post design** is a weaker design that compares the intervention group to itself at baseline. Both these designs are improved by collecting data again a few weeks or months after the conclusion of the intervention, to establish two postintervention data collection points. The second data collection point demonstrates whether changes that were seen as a result of the intervention are sustained over at least the brief period of time between the end of the intervention and the third data collection. These designs are referred to as two-group/pre-post-post and one-group/pre-post-post designs. Many good books detailing research designs are available, and it is advisable to consult one while planning the evaluation (Shadish, Cook, & Campbell, 2002).

An outcome evaluation determines whether the overall goals of the intervention were met. In reality, the ultimate outcome of most community-based health interventions cannot be assessed because of the limited time and resources available or because of limited statistical power. For example, if the overall goal of an intervention implemented in one of two churches is to improve the cardiac health of women through increased levels of physical activity, the impact evaluation may assess changes in women's cardiovascular mortality rates. Detecting such a change, however, will be very difficult considering the amount of time that would be needed to examine this outcome. In addition, other extraneous factors—such as improvements in medical technology and diagnosis—can also contribute to a decrease in mortality rates, making it difficult to determine how much of the change is ultimately due to the intervention.

Step 4: Selecting Reliable Indicators

Indicators to measure the success of the intervention must be selected for each specific objective. Several factors go into the selection of indicators or variables to measure intervention success, including the availability of data, the unit of analysis, and the **reliability** of the indicator.

The availability of measures and the difficulty in collecting them should be thought through in this selection process. For example, in an intervention with the overall aim of decreasing adolescent pregnancies and the specific objective of implementing a communitywide after-school sports intervention, it may be feasible to follow a cohort of participants using a **prospective cohort design.** If this is the case, data could be collected on the number of pregnancies and perhaps compared to a similar population not exposed to the intervention. In small-scale or pilot projects, however, such a design is seldom possible. More common is a one-year intervention where it will not be possible to use the communitywide adolescent rate as an indicator because there is a time lag in the availability of these rates. If the intervention is being implemented at the level of only one school district or in one or two individual schools, overall adolescent pregnancy rates are generally not available at that level of measurement. This is where knowledge of the literature can provide alternative measures of intervention impact, such as changes in grades or plans for the future or attitudes about pregnancy.

The evaluation plan should include an ecological unit of analysis. In other words, all analysis related to the evaluation must occur at the individual, organization, or community level (see Chapter Four). Evaluations that analyze at the organization and community level are more robust than those that use individual- or group-level measures, because an intervention that is being implemented in only one setting—say, one school or one church—can be analyzed only at the individual level. If access to several schools or churches is possible, however, analysis can occur at both the individual and the aggregate school or church level. The sample size and thus statistical power become issues here, so a statistician will need to be consulted.

The strength of the indicators in terms of predicting an outcome is an important consideration. In interventions at the ecological levels of group, organization, and system, change at the level of knowledge is a commonly used but a relatively weak indicator of effectiveness, because in general a change in knowledge has little effect on a change in behavior. Stronger indicators than knowledge that can be used to assess intervention effectiveness are changes in attitudes, including self-efficacy; skills; behaviors; and the strongest indicator: health indices (Kirkpatrick & Kirkpatrick, 2006). All health interventions should at least measure change in knowledge and attitudes. Measuring changes in skills is a stronger indicator of behavior change and the best indicator of an intervention's success. While ideally the goal of every community-based health intervention is change and improvement in communitywide indices (that is, morbidity and mortality statistics), for short-term interventions this is generally not feasible because of the time lag in the availability of such data.

An example of these levels can be seen in an intervention to improve the health of children with asthma in a specific geographic community—an intervention at the ecological level of group. The overall goal might be to decrease asthma-related mortality and the specific objectives to decrease asthma-related hospitalizations and emergency room visits, with intervention-related activities offered to children diagnosed with asthma attending all elementary and middle schools of the district. While it may be theoretically possible to actually collect baseline and follow-up data about asthma-related emergency room visits in the community's hospitals and urgent care centers, Health Insurance Portability and Accountability Act (HIPAA) regulations generally make this form of data difficult to impossible to collect, unless the practitioner is a member of the hospital or care center staff; it would also be necessary to collect these data from each hospital or care center, since intervention activities could result in changes in the number of visits at one institution and not at the other.

If collection of such communitywide health indices is not feasible, however, data can be collected on several other indicators. In addition to knowledge and attitudes about asthma care and prevention, demonstration of correct inhaler use (skills) before and after the intervention is usually feasible. It might also be possible for the evaluation team to return three to six months after the intervention and collect data on the number of emergency room and urgent care center visits (behaviors) that occurred in the interim. Of course, baseline data on the number of such visits should also be collected in the interval before the start of the intervention. This asthma-related intervention would therefore assess change in knowledge, attitudes, and skills related to asthma care as well as behaviors, all varied and strong indicators of intervention success.

FLEXIBILITY: AN ESSENTIAL SKILL IN EVALUATION

In implementing both the intervention and the evaluation, the practitioner must be able to maintain flexibility. Many things can go wrong, and some undoubtedly will. Policy makers or public officials may object to some aspect of the evaluation design, people may object to being interviewed, an organization may drop out before the intervention is complete, or people may drop out before follow-up data are collected. Viable alternatives are almost always available, though they may not be readily apparent. For example, staff members might be available to be interviewed rather than their supervisors. The sample size can be increased to make up for dropouts, and additional subjects may be recruited at the remaining organizations. In the worst-case scenario, the planned evaluation design may need to be rethought to make the best use of the data that are available.

SUMMARY

This chapter provided the reader with the rationale for and steps of an evaluation which every intervention should contain. Distinctions between the three types of evaluation were made, as well as specifications about when to use process, impact, and outcome evaluation. The reader should now be familiar with the basics of the different types of evaluation methodologies and the data used in those methodologies. The chapter concluded with strategies for disseminating both positive and negative evaluation results.

KEY TERMS

Baseline data

Control group

Experimental group

Fidelity

Gantt chart

Impact evaluation

Outcome evaluation

Placebo

Pre-post design

Process evaluation

Prospective cohort design

Qualitative methods

Quantitative methods

Quasi-experimental designs

Randomized-controlled trial

Reliability

Semistructured interviews

Statistical significance

Triangulation of methods

Two-group/pre-post design

Unit of analysis

ACTIVITIES

1. Describe three outcome and three process objectives for an intervention to reduce tobacco use among teenage girls in the three high schools of a district.

2. The launch of Gardisil, the first cervical cancer vaccine that protects against four types of human papillomavirus (HPV), was followed by the implementation of policies and programs to increase awareness and ensure that those who wanted to receive the vaccine (and were within the recommended age range) would have access. If you were designing an evaluation to accompany a new intervention aimed at increasing awareness among residents in rural Nebraska, how would you prospectively plan for an outcome evaluation? What might some of the evaluable objectives be for this intervention? Write these down and identify which methods-—interviews, surveys, or others—you would use to evaluate the objectives and why.

DISCUSSION QUESTION

1. What triangulation methods might be used to evaluate a community-based after-school intervention with an overall aim of decreasing substance abuse among thirteen- to seventeen-year-olds?

4

LEARNING FROM THE PAST AND ADAPTING TO THE FUTURE

FUNDING AND SUSTAINABILITY

LEARNING OBJECTIVES

- Understand the differences between the major sources of funding
- Become familiar with strategies to identify potential funding opportunities from both government and private sources
- Appreciate the importance and challenge of sustaining an intervention

OVERVIEW

Almost all interventions need funding for both their initial implementation and their continuation. This chapter presents an overview of ways to seek funding for a health intervention, along with organizational and political strategies to increase an intervention's potential for continuation into the foreseeable future.

FINANCING COMMUNITY-BASED HEALTH INTERVENTIONS

Unless financial support is available to the practitioner as an employee of an agency that funds its own interventions, such as a local health department, it will be necessary to seek external funding. Interventions can be funded with public funds allocated by federal or local governmental agencies or privately, through foundation funding. Grants are sources of money that are awarded by government agencies (federal, state, and local) and philanthropic foundations to recipients for the purpose of carrying out a project that supports and promotes the public good. Typically, grants are awarded to organizations and not individuals, although the individuals who are named as key personnel when the grant proposal is submitted will be in charge of the work. Grants are seldom available to individuals who are not applying through an established organization.

Almost all grants are awarded through a formal application process, with eligibility requirements, application forms, deadline dates, and procedures varying for each funding agency. It is important to understand the requirements and other information associated with the particular agency from which funding will be requested. This information is available at a local or regional foundation library or at the office of sponsored programs in an academic institution. Internet search engines can point you to information warehouses that collect, store, and provide information on grant opportunities. The federal government's web site can be used to search for government grants (www.grants.gov), and the Foundation Center offers useful information on philanthropic grant opportunities (www.foundationcenter.org).

Potential Sources of Funding

1. *Government Agencies.* Federal, state, and local government agencies regularly publish requests for proposals (RFPs) or requests for applications (RFAs). The National Institute on Drug Abuse and the National Institute of Mental Health, both of which are parts of the National Institutes of Health, and the New York State Department of Health are a few examples. Submissions of proposals are generally solicited within a specified time period. Following the submission period, all proposals are reviewed by committees of reviewers who are experts in the topic area. The committee members score the proposals and select those graded as methodologically sound and closest to the intent of the request for proposals. The application process for funds from grantmaking institutions tends to be time-consuming and complicated and calls for a

sophisticated understanding of research methodology and budgeting. Although tedious, this process also offers the potential for substantial funding awards.

2. *Philanthropic Foundations*. Philanthropic foundations award grant dollars nationally and internationally to support the public good. Initial proposals to foundations tend to be less formal and complex than those to government agencies. Foundations have distinct areas of interest that allow researchers and practitioners to match their interests with those of the foundation. Other than a few large exceptions such as Gates, Rockefeller, and Robert Wood Johnson, foundations generally award relatively small amounts of money compared to government awards.

Philanthropic private foundations are nongovernmental, nonprofit organizations whose funds generally come from a principal endowment. Foundation budgets are typically managed by their own trustees and directors. They are also most likely to fund projects within their local geographic area or community. For example, the Fund for the City of New York is interested only in projects that are undertaken in New York City, the Missouri Health Care Foundation funds projects in central and eastern Missouri, and the Stuart Family Foundation works in the San Francisco Bay area. If it is interested in a specific project, a foundation may offer to assist in the development of a fundable proposal.

Following are some of the different types of philanthropic foundations:

- **Independent or family foundations** receive endowments from individuals or families; family foundations tend to have significant donor or donor-family involvement

- **Operating foundations** run their own programs and services and typically do not provide much grant support to outside organizations

- **Community foundations** seek support from the public, but like private foundations they provide grants; their grants primarily support the needs of the geographic community or region in which they are located

- **Other public foundations** include funds serving other population groups and field-specific funds such as women's funds and health funding foundations set up with proceeds from the sale of nonprofit health care facilities, also called conversion funds or new health foundations (Foundation Center, 2009)

3. *Corporate Foundations*. Corporate foundations are distinct from government and nonprofit foundations because they are run by for-profit companies that offer corporate giving programs. These foundations are legally separate entities from their parent companies, which are the source of their funds, but the budgets are typically managed by corporate staff members (Foundation Center, 2009). Examples of corporate giving programs include Verizon, Bank of America, American Century, and most of the large pharmaceutical companies.

Eligibility for Funding

Generally speaking, four types of groups are eligible to apply for grants:

1. Government organizations
   - State governments
   - Local governments
   - City or township governments
   - Special district governments
   - Native American tribal governments

2. Education organizations
   - Independent school districts
   - Public and state-controlled institutions of higher education
   - Private institutions of higher education

3. Public housing organizations
   - Public housing authorities
   - Native American housing authorities

4. Nonprofit organizations
   - Nonprofits that have established 501(c)(3) status with the IRS, other than institutions of higher education (www.grants.gov/aboutgrants/eligibility.jsp)

At times nonprofit agencies that have not yet received legal recognition of their nonprofit status from the state will apply for funding through another community non-profit agency that has this status and pay the lead agency a small percentage of the funds for this service.

The Difference Between Contracts and Grants

Some government agencies like the Centers for Disease Control and Prevention tend to offer contracts rather than grants. The main difference between grants and contracts largely concerns reporting to the agency. Funding agencies that provide contracts have more stringent reporting requirements and supervise their grantees more closely than grantmaking agencies, which only require periodic progress reports. Not adhering to contract reporting requirements can result in the withdrawal of the remaining funds. The grantee's responsibility in a federal grant is to produce findings that can be dis-seminated at the end of the funding period in a form such as reports and peer-reviewed published manuscripts. Not following through on dissemination makes it less likely for federal agencies to award funding in future.

Selecting Potential Funders

When allocating grant dollars, funders base their decisions on the fit of their mission with the activities and intervention described in a proposal. Time is well spent learning about the mission and goals of the government agency and foundation to which a proposal could potentially be sent. Go to the web sites of the funding agencies and study grantee awards made over the past few years. Try to identify an agency whose mission matches closely with the activities proposed in your intervention. The match can be the location or city where the work is being done, the target population, or the problem that the intervention will address. Knowing a funder's giving trends can help focus a proposal for funding.

Examine the number and size of awards given to past recipients, so that the requested amount is within the limits that the funder is likely to consider. Initial requests for funding are more likely to be granted if the requests are for moderate amounts of money—that is, under $10,000. Demonstrating competence and success in delivering what is promised in a proposal will strengthen the reputation of both the agency and the practitioner and enhance the chances for future funding in larger amounts.

After you have identified potential funders, download and carefully review the organization's instructions and invitation to submit a proposal, also known as a **request for proposals** (RFPs) or **request for applications** (RFAs). These materials provide detailed instructions on the various components required for the application and how to complete the forms attached to the instructions. Review these materials before beginning to write and carefully note specifications on page limits, margins, font sizes, and allowable appendixes. Specifications about available funds and insight into reviewers' criteria will generally be provided. Look for the resources that are provided to applicants; many funding organizations offer teleconferences or web conferences as well as contact information on organizational representatives who will answer questions or provide further information on the proposal. These resources will help determine whether a project is potentially eligible for funding or whether it would need to be modified to meet the organization's funding criteria.

COMPONENTS OF THE PROPOSAL FOR FUNDING

Since the due dates for the submission of proposals are fixed, good planning is necessary to gather and complete all the parts. Writing a proposal is hard work and it helps to break the task into component parts and develop a work plan to stay on track. Remember that the proposal will probably have to be reviewed by the university or applying agency's budget office before submission; these offices generally require at least a day or two to approve a proposal. If, for example, an application is due on March 1, which happens to fall on a Monday, the applying agency's approving offices will need lead time to review it, so the application must be completed at some point in the preceding week—probably Wednesday, February 24, at the latest. This reality comes as a surprise to many novice grant writers, so incorporating this information into the work plan will save considerable last-minute stress and ensure that deadlines are met.

The application processes of funding agencies vary, with some requesting that applicants submit a **letter of intent** before the date of the full proposal. Generally, this letter is simply a written statement expressing the intention to apply for funding; however, some agencies request that a letter of intent include a brief summary of the elements in a full grant proposal. The letter of intent must be thorough, clear, and concise and follow the format identified in the grant announcement.

Funders also have different requirements as to the degree of specificity of the proposed intervention. The National Institutes of Health generally outline a problem area, but leave the nature of the intervention up to the researcher or practitioner, allowing a great deal of latitude in designing the intervention. The Centers for Disease Control and Prevention often have a specific intervention in mind and publish a RFP or RFA detailing the programmatic activities that must be undertaken by the grantee within a specific period of time. Foundations may have a shifting focus area, with general calls for interventions on obesity in one funding cycle and mental health in another; in these cases the intervention content can usually be determined by the applicant.

The Proposal Abstract

While the structure of a funding proposal varies, most will include the following material, either in discrete sections or as part of the general information. The **abstract** of a proposal will often have a specific word or space limit and is a clear and concise summary of the proposal's aims, objectives, and methodology. Three examples of funding abstracts are provied on the present page through page 147.

Proposal Abstract: Example 1

The proposed research project will test an innovative model to address excess rates of family violence in two Native American communities. Researchers will draw on the strengths of these communities and work with an existing women's council to attain the goal of decreasing the incidence of family violence and increase the ability of the communities to carry out future projects. This community-academic partnership, Grandmothers as a Community Resource to Decrease Family Violence, will work with elders and the Council of Women to jointly conduct all aspects of the proposed project and answer the following four research questions:

1. How does the intervention and its activities affect family violence statistics in the targeted communities? How does the intervention affect violence-related community activities?

2. Can intervention activities change attitudes about the social acceptability of family violence and increase self-efficacy among individuals and families participating in intervention activities?

3. Do intervention activities change attitudes about violence and increase collective efficacy and social capital in the communities?

4. What are the community barriers to and facilitators of training grandmothers to implement community-based participatory research methods in Native American communities?

Researchers will work with the existing Council of Women to expand its membership to include grandmothers and work with the tribal councils of the Prairie Band Pottawatomie and the Kickapoo communities. Together they will select and implement individual-, family-, and community-level programs to change attitudes toward violence and improve prevention efficacy among women and children. Intervention activities will be based on both social cognitive theory and cultural practices and beliefs unique to each tribe. Programming with individuals, families, and the larger community will remain in place for a period of three years. Multilevel outcome variables will include violence-related statistics; community engagement as measured by key informant interviews and by a pre- and post intervention survey on violence attitudes and social capital in the two communities; family violence attitudes, skills, and behaviors of grandmothers and women trained as interventionists; and family violence prevention attitudes, skills, and behaviors of community women and children participating in the intervention programs. The Council of Women and the grandmothers will work side by side with researchers in the data collection and analysis process and share responsibility for dissemination of outcomes in community and academic venues.

Proposal Abstract: Example 2

The intervention is based on diffusion of innovations theory and will involve training carefully selected student opinion leaders to change social norms and reduce HIV/AIDS risk behavior among their school peers. Opinion leader interventions will identify and educate influential members of a community to catalyze changes in social norms within the leaders' social networks and eventually in the community at large. The project will apply this intervention model to an adolescent population in Cape Town, South Africa. Tenth graders who have been identified as opinion leaders in their school-based social networks will be recruited and trained with skills to influence

(Continued)

(*Continued*)

their peers (predominantly through informal social contact). The training program will include role-playing and interactive exercises and will run from the summer break between tenth and eleventh grade into the students' eleventh-grade year. Conducting the research among older high school students is preferable for evaluating the intervention because a greater number of older students are sexually active, enabling assessment of the effects of the intervention on condom use.

To assess the effectiveness of this intervention, an anonymous survey of the eleventh graders will be undertaken in intervention and control schools at baseline (the beginning of the school year), five months later, and again nine months after the baseline survey at completion of the intervention and close of the school year. The study will investigate the effects of the intervention on the following outcomes:

1. Delay the onset of sexual activity among those not sexually active at baseline

2. Increase safe sexual practices in students who have had sexual intercourse, including an increase in the use of condoms, a decrease in the number of sexual partners, and a decrease in sexual coercion and violence

3. Affect the proposed mechanism for behavior change: perceptions of social or normative pressures about the acceptance of unprotected sexual intercourse and gender violence

4. Improve students' attitudes and reduce stigmatization of those infected with HIV/AIDS

5. Improve students' knowledge about HIV/AIDS transmission, and reduce misinformation about HIV/AIDS and condoms

Proposal Abstract: Example 3

The overarching goal of the Healthy Living project is to improve cardiovascular and respiratory health conditions affected by environmental and behavioral factors in the urban core of Any Town, USA. Following are the project objectives:

1. To increase public awareness and knowledge about overweight, obesity, cardiovascular health, respiratory health, and asthma

2. To address environmental factors in the home that contribute to overweight, obesity, heart disease, stroke, and asthma

3. To address environmental factors in the community that contribute to obesity, heart disease, stroke, and asthma

4. To increase resources for faith-based organizations and community-based organizations so that they can better serve the target population and address the identified health problems

5. To empower a group of youth advocates to work in the community to reduce the incidence of obesity, heart disease, stroke, and asthma through an extensive social marketing campaign targeting Any Town that will be compared with Other Town, which has a similar population

The **specific aims** section generally contains a brief description of the problem to be addressed, the overall goal and specific aims of the proposed intervention, and a brief description of the methods that will be used. This section may repeat parts of the abstract, but it contains additional detail about both the problem and the method.

The **background and significance** section presents the writer's knowledge about the problem, its incidence in the community, and the current health literature about interventions and about the target population. This section should conclude with a few sentences about how the proposed intervention will help address the problem or meet the described community health need.

The **methods** or **methodology** section is generally the most carefully reviewed part of a grant application. This is the place to describe in detail how the proposed intervention will be carried out. The specifics of the intervention or curriculum should be included, along with how, where, and when the activities will take place and who will deliver and receive the intervention. This information should be presented in a way that allows a reader who is completely unfamiliar with the health problem and the community to clearly understand how grant funds will be used. Jargon should be avoided and all abbreviations spelled out the first time they are used.

Include an **evaluation** plan, either as a stand-alone section or as part of the methods section. Even if the intervention is not research in the formal sense, this plan should describe how intervention activities will be monitored, what the desired outcomes are, and how success will be determined (see Chapter Ten for further information on evaluations).

Most funding agencies want to know about the background and skills of the person(s) who will carry out the intervention (the project manager or principal investigator). Agencies also want to see a demonstration of the **organizational capacity** to complete the project and provide implementation support. The organization capacity section should also include at least a few sentences documenting the background and skills of the principal investigator or project manager. This information is not offered for the purpose of bragging or self-aggrandizement; it is provided to inform the funding agency that personnel and organization skills are available to successfully complete the proposed intervention. Organizational capacity also necessitates the gathering of background information describing the applicant organization. At a college or university, this is often called **boilerplate information** and describes the facilities, library, computer support, and financial administration of grant funds. If the applicant is a community organization, the information should include a brief history of the agency, the mission and goals, the organizational chart, description of the board of directors, and a brief account of current or previous programs. Often documentation of nonprofit status is also required.

Sample University Boilerplate Information

XYZ University has provided teaching, research, and service to state residents since 1839. Today the university is one of the nation's largest and most prestigious public research universities, with more than 100,000 students on four campus locations and hundreds of thousands served statewide through University Extension. The university has both graduate and undergraduate programs, with faculty conducting a wide variety of research and community-based service projects.

All faculty and staff have Pentium-based personal computers in their offices with up-to-date software necessary to support research projects, including qualitative and quantitative data analysis programs. Access to office computers and files is available 24/7 through VPN and Virtual Desktop programs. Faculty offices are equipped with telephones that have conference call capability. Equipment for video conferences through PolyCom is available at several locations throughout the university to allow audiovisual communication with multiple distant sites.

The university libraries inspire scholarship by evaluating, collecting, organizing, preserving, and creating access to sources of knowledge through effective and innovative service delivery. The university libraries are an essential information resource for the entire community. The collection covers the information needs of medicine, nursing, public health, and pharmacy researchers. Current and comprehensive library holdings are available both on-campus and through electronic access. The library holds 1,621,038 volumes; more than 6,839 serial subscriptions (542 e-journals); more than 1.9 million pieces of microfilm; over 362,758 sound recordings, and 3,811 films and videos. The library provides online access to computerized databases including MEDLINE, CINAHL, UM, OVID databases, EBSCO, OCLC FirstSearch, RLIN/BIB, MOBIUS and MIRACL. These databases can be accessed both in the library and remotely via the Internet. Many journals offer full-text articles online.

XYZ University provides the intervention team with the infrastructure necessary to carry out the proposed intervention. Physical space for research assistance, storage space for data, computer hardware, statistical programs and technical support for analysis, and staff for management of grant finances and preparation and submission of reports and manuscripts are all easily available. XYZ University has the experience and infrastructure to administer and manage multiple, diverse funding awards. From preaward support to postaward administration and research protections, the Office of Research Services is a key element in the university's research infrastructure. This infrastructure has experience with the rapid implementation of new projects through the establishment of PeopleSoft accounts, monthly financial reports, and multiple subcontracts.

If other agencies are involved, a letter from them outlining their specific contribution, expertise, and support is needed. Individuals outside the applicant agency who will be involved with the intervention should also provide a résumé and a **letter of collaboration** describing how their expertise will contribute to the intervention.

Sample Description of Background and Skills of Staff

Maria Gonzalez, the coordinator for the proposed intervention, is a graduate student in public health at XYZ University. She received her BA degree from State University where she was a regular volunteer at the adolescent drop-in shelter. She currently juggles her class work with a part-time job as a production assistant at National Studios.

Stan Jones, assistant coordinator for the proposed intervention, has worked as the special programs director at the Neighborhood Arts Council for the past five years. In addition to his work with elementary school students and senior citizens, he developed and successfully implemented the PhotoVoice program with youth on probation from the juvenile justice system (described fully in news article in Appendix III).

David Stephens, the evaluation consultant for the proposed intervention, is an associate professor in the Department of Community Health in XYZ University. He has conducted process, outcome, and impact evaluations for a variety of community-based programs, most recently the Dramatic AIDS Education Project, and the Healthy Hearts/Healthy Kids symposium.

Sample Letter of Collaboration

Maria Gonzalez
XYZ University
2220 Main Street
Any Town, USA 12345
[Date]
Dear Ms. Gonzalez:

As the director of the St. Thomas Day Care Center, which serves children and families in the urban core of our community, I know firsthand the terrible impact that violence has had on their lives. We are very excited about working with you and your intervention research team on the development and implementation of violence prevention programs with the families of our center. I believe your ideas about working together with staff, parents, and young people are excellent and will reap many benefits, both in terms of skills acquisition and in lowering the rate of violence-related problems.

Specifically, we will allow you to implement your STOP the Violence intervention with our staff, our families, and our children during the upcoming school year. We wish you every success in achieving funding in this important area.

Sincerely,
Jose Charles
Director

COMPONENTS OF THE BUDGET

The **budget** can simply describe the expected expenses or can give more detail on the expenses that will be incurred during the funding period, the **in-kind** or nonmonetary support that will be tapped, and any revenue that may be generated. The funder will generally specify a format and guidelines to be used to develop the budget pages. The budget should be specific, realistic, and should offer the grant reviewer a snapshot of what is being proposed. Try to make the budgeted amounts as realistic as possible and not wild estimates. Accompanying the budget should be a **budget justification**, a narrative statement that describes the need for each of the items that have been budgeted. For example, if an interviewer is required to interview twenty respondents, and each interview will take half a day including travel, the budget justification would indicate the need for ten days of interviewing by an interviewer who will be hired at $XX per day.

Personnel and OTPS

A simple budget looks at expenses in two categories: **personnel** and **other than personnel services (OTPS)**. The personnel section includes two items: staff members' salaries and benefits. When identifying needed intervention personnel, consider how many and what types of personnel are realistically needed. How much of the executive director's time will be required? Will a full-time project manager be required? Is an outside consultant needed for technical or professional expertise? Will administrative or secretarial help be necessary? Will the evaluation be conducted by someone on the project or will a subcontract be offered to an outside evaluator? What percentage of time will each staff person spend on the project—that is, will they be full-time or part-time? If part-time, for exactly what percentage of full-time will they be hired?

Fringe benefits include mandated expenses such as Social Security, worker's compensation insurance, and state unemployment insurance and voluntary benefits such as health insurance and retirement programs. These benefits are expressed as a percentage of each salary—for example, "15 percent of the project director's $30,000 annual salary, or $4,500," with the percentage determined by the payroll or budget office. Salaries and fringe benefits should be listed as separate items in the personnel category.

The OTPS section of the budget identifies all the expenses that are non-personnel-related. The equipment category includes items such as a computer, statistical software, a printer, and other intervention-related equipment such as pedometers, scales, and blood-pressure cuffs. The consumables or supplies category includes office supplies such as stationery, pens, pencils, copying supplies such as toner and paper, and expenses such as printing and publicity. Intervention-related supplies like participant workbooks and incentives such as movie tickets, grocery vouchers, and bookstore gift cards are listed in this section.

Travel expenses should be estimated and include local and national travel. Estimate the amount that staff will spend on intervention-related travel such as site visits and include a line item for local mileage, gas, and public transit fares. If out-of-town travel is anticipated, such as travel to professional meetings to disseminate results, include air or train travel expenses, accommodations, registration fees, and a per diem food allowance. Finally, for items that do not fit into another category, an **other expenses** category can include miscellaneous costs such as postage, advertising, subscriptions, and small intervention-related costs.

The Budget Justification

An example of a budget justification appears in Table 11.1.

Indirect Costs

Institutions and most organizations charge funders a set amount of money for indirect costs, also referred to as overhead. This is calculated as a percentage of the personnel

TABLE 11.1   **Example of budget justification for HIV prevention intervention: twelve-month period**

Personnel	Amount	Justification and Responsibilities
Maria Gonzalez	$ 8,000	20% full-time equivalent × $40,000 annual salary = $8,000
Coordinator		Responsible for overall implementation of all aspects of project and securing IRB approval, hiring, training, and supervision of staff and volunteers. Collaborate in data analysis and writing of reports and manuscripts and copresent at professional meetings.
Fringe on Smith	$ 2,667	Fringe rate of 33% × $8,000 = $2,667
Stan Jones	$ 15,000	50% full-time equivalent × $30,000 annual salary = $15,000
Assistant coordinator		Responsible for recruiting and training adolescents from target group to implement video production, arranging venues for dissemination of completed video, and assisting in data collection for evaluation.
Fringe on Jones	$ 5,000	Fringe rate of 33% × $15,000 = $5,000
David Stephens	$ 2,500	consultant
		Responsible for development and implementation of all aspects of evaluation
Total Personnel	**$ 30,667**	

Other Than Personnel

Item	Amount	Description
Payment for adolescent filmmakers	$ 2,400	10 adolescents × 10 hours @ $12/hour = $1,200 5 adolescents × 20 hours @ $12/hour = $1,200 Adolescent filmmakers, who will be identified through liaisons with public housing office
Transportation to presentations	$ 105	10 presentations × 30 miles per presentation trip = 300 miles @ .35/mile = $105
Rental of video equipment	$ 520	Camera, lights, splicer for 8 weeks @ $65/week = $520
Video supplies	$ 200	Estimated at $200
Refreshments at presentations	$ 750	$75 for refreshments × 10 presentations = $750
Conference travel	$ 630	For dissemination at state public health association conference; includes $150 registration fee, hotel for 2 nights @ $120/night = $240, meals for 3 days @ $45 per diem rate = $135, and round-trip mileage to conference, 300 miles × .35/mile = $105
Office supplies	$ 250	Paper and ink cartridges for the project coordinator's activities
Total Other Than Personnel	**$ 4,855**	
GRAND TOTAL	**$35,522**	

cost, and it is used to pay for things like space, electricity, access to libraries, and so forth. Federal agencies like the NIH commonly pay universities over 50 percent of the personnel costs as overhead. Foundations pay usually between 10 and 15 percent. The applicant generally does not need to include these costs as part of the budget, as they will be calculated after the grant is awarded.

Grant Writing Tips for Beginners

For initial grantseeking attempts, applications to smaller local foundations are a good place to start. Project officers may be willing to read drafts of a proposal before final submission. Building relationships with the staff members of a small private foundation will often pay off in future endeavors.

Consider working with an experienced grant writer who will read over the grant proposal and provide suggestions or assist in putting the overall proposal together. Taking a course on grant writing, often available through a local community college or university, provides a chance to both learn these basics and have a draft reviewed by objective readers before submitting for funding. Such training is also available online at the Foundation Center's web site: http://foundationcenter.org/getstarted/training/online.

New or developing community-based organizations that are not yet incorporated or do not yet have official nonprofit status can apply for grants by using another agency as a **fiscal agent.** This strategic alliance achieves mutually beneficial outcomes by allowing a new group to receive grant dollars that they may not have been eligible for otherwise. The lead agency generally receives about 1 percent of the award for managing the grant budget.

If the total budget for the proposed intervention exceeds the amount that can be obtained from one funding agency, it is possible to request funding for a distinct part of a proposal such as training and stipends for peer educators or salary for a half-time coordinator. After receiving a commitment for even a small amount of money, it is easier to go to other funders and request their collaboration in the intervention activities. Many larger foundations allow project officers to award small discretionary grants—generally below $25,000—without requiring approval of the foundation's entire board, which may meet only once or twice a year. Remember, however, that foundations like to be able to show in their annual reports what they have accomplished through their funding, so divide the budget and requests into distinct intervention categories. For example, rather than splitting the total expenses of the budget for an adolescent HIV prevention intervention, ask one foundation for funding for the adolescent videotaping component of the intervention and another for funding travel and dissemination of the videotape. This allows both funding agencies to report concrete support for the intervention. For further information, refer to texts written by Brown and Brown (2001), Browning (2008), Carlson (2002), and Karsh and Fox (2003).

CONTINUING AND SUSTAINING AN INTERVENTION

The implementation of a successful community health intervention does not provide any guarantee of its continuation beyond the end of the original funding period. Few funders will support an intervention indefinitely, so new resources must be identified to enable continuation of intervention activities. Developing a plan for sustainability or continuation should be a goal for all successful interventions.

While minimal research has been conducted on sustainability, there is agreement on several activities that can increase the likelihood of an intervention's sustainability (Scheirer, 2005). A good fit between an intervention and a community agency's culture and mission will increase the likelihood that the agency can integrate the intervention into its core functioning. An intervention can be more easily sustained if it works well within the existing organizational climate of the community agency and its existing resources than an intervention that requires considerable additional resources or a change in the organizational climate or structure.

Gaining the support of people in the organization's administration before starting the intervention is critical for continuation. A staff member at the administrative level can be an excellent internal champion and assist in both intervention implementation and sustainability. Emphasize the benefits of the intervention to achieve buy-in from staff members, clients, and other stakeholders. Be prepared to clearly demonstrate these benefits and their congruence with both the agency and the funder's missions. If agency staff members are needed to make the intervention work, intervention responsibilities should overlap with the general area of their current job responsibilities and should be easy to integrate into daily routines. Staff should not have to neglect their job responsibilities to participate in intervention tasks (Scheirer, 2005).

SUMMARY

This chapter focused on some of the specifics involved in acquiring funding for proposed intervention projects. It discussed how and where to apply for funds, and the differences between applying for government versus private funds. The chapter included a discussion of the components of a grant proposal, along with recommended ways to present a budget. Ideas for sustaining an intervention after receiving initial funding were also presented.

KEY TERMS

Abstract
Background and significance
Boilerplate information
Budget
Budget justification
Evaluation
Fiscal agent
Fringe benefits
In-kind
Letter of collaboration

Letter of intent
Methods or methodology
Organizational capacity
Other expenses
Other than personnel services (OTPS)
Personnel
Request for applications (RFAs)
Request for proposals (RFPs)
Specific aims

ACTIVITIES

1. Identify one foundation that funds health interventions in your community and describe at least three interventions that they funded last year.

2. Locate their funding application and due dates for the upcoming year or grant cycle.

3. Give two reasons why this foundation should fund your intervention.

DISCUSSION QUESTIONS

1. Discuss the pros and cons of applying for foundation funds versus federal funds to support an intervention.

2. Is one type more appropriate than the other for specific types of projects?

CHAPTER

IMPLEMENTATION PITFALLS

LEARNING OBJECTIVES

- Enumerate three common areas in which implementation problems tend to occur in community-based interventions
- Become familiar with strategies to overcome pitfalls as they occur during a community-based intervention

OVERVIEW

This chapter reviews several problems that practitioners often encounter as they implement their interventions.

THINGS HAPPEN

Even with the basic guidance provided in this book on implementing a community-based health intervention, it is important to recognize that many things can go wrong. While this is certainly true in all health and research projects, community settings present a special challenge because of the myriad of relationships that must be successfully negotiated. Issues arise that simply could not be anticipated. The key to success is to be able to think through and respond to difficult situations in a timely and effective manner. No matter what an initial personal reaction might be, the appropriate professional response is to remain calm and review the whole picture before reacting. This whole-picture approach requires addressing the problem that has come up while minimizing the impact on the intervention's goals, methodology, and scientific integrity. Maintaining this balance is an optimal way to maximize both community satisfaction and scientific results.

Pitfalls can appear in the design, the implementation, or the evaluation stage of an intervention. In this chapter we have pulled together some real-life examples from our own experiences.

Design Pitfalls

Underestimating the time and resources to complete a project is a common pitfall, especially for students eager to help a community change a health problem. Be realistic about your budget and avoid squeezing the budget for a larger project into the confines of a smaller one. Think through the many tasks involved in seeing the intervention through from start to finish by detailing the many tasks that are involved, and educate funders and agency staff early about these tasks. Include mechanisms in the plan that will ensure that planning activities are on track. For example, make a timeline for the project and discuss it with the funders and agency staff (see Chapter Nine). Another way to stay on track is to hold biweekly staff meetings to examine progress and make adjustments as necessary. This also helps to produce quarterly reports on the activities and progress. Some funding agencies may require this, and even if they do not, such reports can prove useful for writing up results after the intervention has been completed. Discuss with the staff any problems that have occurred in maintaining the timeline.

Be realistic about the goals of an intervention and remember that behavior changes take time and may be difficult to assess over a short funding period. Try to avoid overpromising the degree of change to expect from the intervention. Select at least some objectives that are likely to change and can be measured over a short period of time, such as shifts in knowledge or even attitudes. Even short-term shifts will demonstrate the positive results that are needed when seeking further funding. Emphasize the ways in which the sets of activities undertaken at the early stages should have "payoff" for the intervention as it unfolds.

When working with community members in developing the intervention, it is necessary to educate people who have not been exposed to research methodology or who do not understand the scientific aspects of research, which are often taken for granted by students and practitioners. For example, the necessity of drawing a random sample of participants or selecting a control group that will not be part of the intervention is not innately obvious and requires careful explanation. It may be necessary to explain why it is not helpful if all the participants in a focus group are friends of the stakeholders or they all share the same views about the outcome of the intervention. Similarly it may be necessary to ensure that staff and community members working on an intervention understand the necessity of collecting data that move beyond personal experiences or at least collect the personal experiences of a broad sample of community members.

Implementation Pitfalls

Major changes in the intervention may be necessary after an intervention has actually been started. A community agency that originally agreed to follow a specific protocol when the project was being developed may discover that this is no longer possible because of a political issue or because they have changed their view of the importance of the project. Regularly broadening the base of support for the intervention by including stakeholders outside a single sector may help address such challenges. To prevent a loss of support for a project, stakeholders need to be kept in the loop with regular phone calls and individual and group meetings, even when they seem to take time and energy away from the core activities of the intervention.

Another issue to consider is participant retention. Participants are likely to stop attending intervention activities if they are hard to access. Avoid this problem by offering to pay any travel expenses and by running program activities at times when most can attend such as after work or school hours and not during holidays. Activities should occur in locations that are easy to get to. While geographic proximity is important, barriers around the site itself should be considered. For instance, a large hospital or federal building can be difficult to navigate if an individual is unfamiliar with its layout or security systems. Similarly, if participants drive to the site, ensure that parking is available, preferably at no cost.

Another common problem is the practice of relying heavily on volunteers to carry out intervention activities. While volunteers can be very helpful, it is important to recognize that these individuals have competing obligations (work, family, and school) that can limit the time they give or can take them away altogether. Clearly, this degree of instability can negatively affect a program's ability to reach its goals. Related to this problem is the fact that a high turnover of people who are perceived as staff can negatively influence program consistency. Furthermore, volunteers, however willing and committed, may not have the requisite skill set needed, and thus appropriate training must be provided, which can drain resources from the intervention.

Staff Turnover

Another complicating factor can arise when there is heavy reliance on one or two staff members while others are not included in the communication and responsibility loop. Such a situation can cause staff turnover and possible discord within the group working on the intervention. Interventions that work with populations of particularly high need, such as the homeless mentally ill or refugees with very minimal resources, may leave staff members frustrated over their inability to make an impact with the resources available and the lack of support for this population from the community at large. The resultant stress, particularly for staff in frontline positions, can easily lead to burnout on the job. Building in adequate time for staff development, varying schedules, developing ways to mix staff responsibilities, and providing regular supervision, guidance, and feedback may help to address this issue. Thinking through what a career ladder might look like for these staff members may also help to preserve talent and experience for the intervention. Think about ways, for instance, that a coordinator position can be created for a staff member who has demonstrated a commitment to frontline work. Identify additional responsibilities that a staff member may be able to take on after some period of time on the job, such as assisting in preparing educational materials, compiling data, assisting with grant writing, or developing new program activities. Communicate such possibilities to newly hired staff early, and work with the partner agency to ensure they can be realized. Staff turnover can be costly to organizations in terms of additional training and orientation for new staff, the burden that falls on existing staff until a position gets filled, and the momentum and relationships lost when someone leaves the team.

Evaluation Pitfalls

Evaluation of a project, while critical to students, faculty, and funders, can be seen as so threatening that occasionally an organization will refuse to cooperate in providing the data needed for the evaluation because they think it will reflect badly on their performance. An initial strategy to address such a situation is to assure the organization that they will not be identified in the evaluation report. If such a commitment cannot be made or is unsuccessful, determine whether data from that organization can be omitted while maintaining the overall design of the evaluation.

In multiagency interventions, cooperating community agencies may sometimes drop out. For example, if a research question is to understand the strengths of slightly different outreach strategies for an HIV prevention program, each of the agencies may be asked to implement a slightly different protocol, with the goal of understanding which strategy is the best. If data from one of the agencies become unavailable, a more limited evaluation comparing the strategy of the agencies that did provide data will still be useful. Sampling frames can usually be adjusted, and one method of collecting data can usually be substituted for another, even if the results will have less statistical power.

Only rarely does a change in cooperating agencies or the community as a whole result in having to pull the plug on an evaluation because of a necessary change in the design. However, difficult as it may be, stopping the evaluation and therefore the intervention altogether should remain an option when it appears that continuation would be a waste of time and resources. Making it clear from the start of a project that a strong evaluation of the intervention is necessary to determine its effect can help to avoid misunderstanding later in the intervention calendar.

Challenges can arise in collecting some types of data needed for administrative or evaluation purposes. A common problem is the objection to certain questions being asked or to the wording of a particular question. Consider ways that such objections can be dealt with without greatly compromising the strength of the results. If the questionnaire wording is found to be offensive by some important segment of the community or by the institutional review board, new wording can be substituted, even if it is less precise. Wording of questions in surveys and other instruments can be changed. To deal with strong objections, specific questions may have to be dropped. For example, if the intervention is to encourage sexually active young people to decrease risky sexual activity, a questionnaire using the slang words that the young people themselves use to describe sexual activity would be preferable because they would be more easily understood. Some adults in the community may object to the use of such words as offensive. Usually a compromise can be reached with the community that will not seriously reduce the effectiveness of the intervention.

In working in a community with several different immigrant groups, ensuring that each group understands the meaning of the instruments, consent forms, and educational materials can be difficult. In such a situation, it is helpful to have a sheet available that allows you to translate words or terms and make them easier for a specific population to understand. In some populations, literacy may be a problem, especially with older immigrants. Asking each participant if they would like to have the questionnaire read aloud, perhaps because they "forgot their glasses," can minimize embarrassment.

Misunderstanding the hierarchy of an immigrant or other community group is a pitfall encountered by many novices to community work. In some groups, women are not permitted to speak to a stranger without a male family member in the room. In others, the adults are dependent on translation from and into English by young family members. This may be the case even when the questions are of an intimate nature. The practitioner must adapt to such situations even if they seem awkward. One option in this situation is to skip questions that might make the respondent uncomfortable, especially if they are not key to the project outcomes.

During a process evaluation, staff members who are being interviewed may feel that their work is being judged and may become suspicious and less than candid in answering questions. Frequent reassurance is necessary that this is not the case and that all data are confidential. Findings may indicate some of the staff are misinterpreting instructions and need to be corrected.

Negative Findings

Some findings could indicate that the community members most at risk are not being reached by the intervention. Other findings could suggest that the intervention, though well executed, is not making much of an impact on the health problem. Findings that indicate any of these situations must be addressed as soon as possible and will likely involve staff retraining, development of a new outreach or recruitment plan, or even early termination of the intervention.

At times stakeholders or community members may not like or feel comfortable with the results of the evaluation of an intervention that they publicly supported. Agency personnel may be concerned about funding for the intervention in light of negative findings, or the findings may not be politically palatable to a segment of the community. Addressing such a situation will depend on whether you plan to continue working with this community. If yes, it may be possible to release findings without showing the community in a negative light by emphasizing positive findings and keeping negative ones out of the public spotlight. A press conference would not be indicated in this situation. However, community members rarely have a problem with publishing negative results in a peer-reviewed journal. In situations when most of the results are positive, holding a press conference in which stakeholders are invited to participate may cement their support for the next stage of work. A press release should always be provided in these situations to guard against misinterpretation or misrepresentation of the findings. When you are disseminating findings, photos can be a good way to visually demonstrate what was done. Remember, however, that authorization must be obtained to use these photos (particularly important if the participants are minors or individuals who may not want to be found, such as injection drug users, undocumented individuals, sexual assault victims, or individuals with criminal records).

If the evaluation has identified some major problems with the intervention, such concerns should be conveyed to the stakeholders to inform them that time and resources could be lost if substantial changes are not instituted. Since bad news can put the messenger in jeopardy, it is best to look to stakeholders who are more likely to understand the nature of research—people experienced with data and evaluation or politically savvy leaders, for example—to help inform those who have not had the same kind of experience.

No intervention unfolds exactly as planned, nor is it likely that the evaluation will be wholly positive. Reporting the findings from an evaluation requires the practitioner to be thoughtful and creative.

SUMMARY

In this chapter we have discussed some of the challenges of working in community settings with numerous relationships that must be successfully negotiated. In our experience, when things go wrong the practitioner must remain calm and think creatively before reacting. The examples presented are by no means an entire inventory of potential pitfalls, but they reflect a range of experiences that can equip readers of this text to manage many of the challenges that lie ahead.

ACTIVITY

1. Construct a list of common pitfalls that might occur in a clinical intervention and a community-based health intervention. How are they similar and how are they different?

DISCUSSION QUESTIONS

1. How would you, as intervention coordinator, respond to learning that your coinvestigator is having a sexual relationship with one of the peer educators in an adolescent pregnancy prevention intervention?

2. What steps can be taken to minimize the falsification of data by data collectors?

THE FUTURE OF COMMUNITY-BASED HEALTH INTERVENTIONS

LEARNING OBJECTIVES

- Envision new methods of community-based health intervention using new methods of communication
- Develop new definitions of *community*, based on the utilization of technological advances

OVERVIEW

This chapter examines the expansion of types of community-based health interventions that are possible with the development of new methods of communication technology.

ADAPTING METHODS OF INTERVENTION TO TWENTY-FIRST–CENTURY COMMUNITIES

The field of public health is constantly in flux. The challenges that we as a society face can change radically in a relatively short period of time. By the middle of the twentieth century, public health practitioners breathed a sigh of relief, believing that many infectious diseases such as smallpox were relics of the past. Polio, which infected over a quarter of a million people in 1988 when the worldwide eradication campaign was started, rapidly became a rare event in the West, although it still claims a number of victims every year in a few communities in South Asia and sub-Saharan Africa where vaccination remains controversial. In 1980, well within living memory, AIDS and HIV had not yet been identified, and public health practitioners felt secure in turning their attention from the prevention of infectious disease to the control and prevention of chronic illnesses such as heart disease and stroke.

By the turn of the twentieth century, however, HIV/AIDS was viewed as a plague that threatened the lives of people on every continent, as millions of people around the world were infected by the virus. Tuberculosis and malaria are still major causes of illness and mortality in parts of the southern hemisphere, and the world remains constantly on guard for the next global pandemic, such as a new and more virulent type of flu. Public health workers must constantly adapt to deal with the new realities of the world in which they work.

Adaptation in public health is not solely about responding to new threats to health. The approaches used to engage with and combat threats to public health and safety must also reflect changes in the way we communicate and interact with those we see as part of our community. One of the major ways that our society and all societies around the world have been changing is in the introduction and adoption of information technologies. In 1980, few people had even heard of the Internet and there were no commercial entities offering access to it. Today billions of people are online. Likewise, the cell phone has moved in a few short decades from a bulky toy for the very wealthy to a sleek common household item. Even in very poor countries and communities, people who cannot afford landline telephone service can purchase a cheap cell phone and the minutes to make necessary calls. These advances in technology have important implications for public health practitioners.

Information Technology Redefines Community

In this chapter, we are moving beyond community as defined and limited by geography to explore how technology has enabled us to think of defining, developing, and reaching communities in all parts of the globe. While access is limited in many vulnerable populations, the penetration of technology continues to spread, especially among the young.

Information technology has altered the definition of *community* in several ways. It has created new and novel communities by connecting people based on shared interests and characteristics regardless of geographic location. While some of these communities are of limited interest for public health purposes, others are extremely relevant. For example, there are online networks of people or communities dedicated to the discussion of everything from pregnancy and weight management to specific diseases and ailments. Other communities form around specific demographic groups, such as women survivors of breast cancer, men who have sex with men, or teenage girls with eating disorders. These communities offer public health workers unique opportunities to observe and interact with specific at-risk populations.

For example, a gay chat room might offer a useful opportunity to observe attitudes and join the conversation about what constitutes risky sexual behavior and then to offer an intervention such as providing facts and evidence on the dangers of unprotected sex. By using the Internet, the practitioner has the ability to answer questions about safe sex and HIV in an environment in which everyone can participate to the extent that they feel comfortable and on an equal footing. This situation could offer the practitioner an opportunity to develop an intervention at a crucial point, ideally *before* people engage in potentially risky behavior, thereby increasing the chance that the information will be salient during the chat or Internet exchange. The advantage of the chat room is that it can reach individuals who are reluctant to participate in a group where they could be identified or feel obligated to reveal information that they wish to keep private. The chat room maintains anonymity for the participants, lowering the barrier of entry below what would be required to attend a meeting, and it avoids the problem of being seen in public picking up potentially embarrassing literature. Questions that may arise while chatting can be easily answered in future contacts through e-mail or other means.

Enhancing Health-Related Communication Through the Internet

The Internet allows public health workers to study the methods of communication, idioms, and slang used by specific groups, which help in crafting messages targeted to the groups in question. The Internet also provides opportunities for the evaluation of the effectiveness of various interventions through various methods such as direct feedback in the form of surveys or indirect feedback in the form of visitation metrics and other statistics.

Paper pamphlets and other conventional forms of health information are distributed without much feedback data on who views them, how they are viewed, and which sections receive the most attention. Web pages offer a new level of targeted marketing with the possibility of an affordable and easy method of collecting responses to the information provided. Webmasters can use computer programs to track how many people visit their sites, how they get to the site, how long they stay, which links they click on, and other information that can be useful in targeting and working with specific communities.

Here is a hypothetical example showing how this can work in the case of an infectious disease. If there is an influenza outbreak in a diverse community with many immigrants, public health officials want to get information out to that community about the precautions people need to take to avoid catching the flu, who is at greatest risk, and how to care for those who become ill. A web page with some basic information can be created in minutes, and it can be dynamically updated minute to minute as additional information comes in. The web site can be presented in a number of languages, with specific instructions targeted to speakers of those languages (such as clinic locations with staff that speak those specific languages). Furthermore, the number of visitors to the web site can be monitored in real time and broken down by language and section for more information.

If the Farsi version of the site is not getting many hits relative to the size of the Farsi-speaking population, this may indicate that more outreach is needed in the Farsi-speaking portion of the community. Likewise, if Spanish speakers are not clicking through to an important section on what to do if a child or older person gets sick, then the page can be redesigned to emphasize links to that section. Information about who is linking to the site can tell the designers which web partners are most effective at driving traffic and which outreach efforts have been most effective. Taken individually, each of these options offers a relatively small advantage, but together they constitute a powerful set of tools for analysis of how well information is being disseminated into various communities or subcommunities.

In another example that is not hypothetical, when health providers see a constellation of illnesses that appear unusual, they can send this information to the local health department or the CDC, which can monitor the number of events to determine whether there is a disease outbreak or potential epidemic and whether an intervention is called for. Health information can be dynamic and quickly changing, and the format of the Internet serves well in such shifting circumstances. In some cases the Internet may offer a unique avenue for disseminating information to or gathering information from people who might otherwise be hard to reach, such as the homebound, those with unusual work hours, or undocumented individuals who are nervous about dealing with anyone in an official capacity.

Using the Internet as a Community Organizing Tool

The Internet also offers opportunities for people to seek information and find communities of people with shared concerns. Popular medical sites like WebMD offer huge amounts of health information that is both easily accessed and potentially useful to a wide variety of people. Every major public health organization, from the American Cancer Society to various smoking cessation campaigns, has a web presence, and their sites offer a variety of services ranging from general background information to detailed plans for sufferers and caregivers to referral services. It is clear that these sites represent valuable new tools in the arsenals of traditional public health organizations, allowing them to expand services and reach people who were previously difficult to inform. We have reached the point where traditional media such as television, print, and even direct mailing advertisements often serve as only a preliminary step and are frequently best used to get people to visit the web sites, which act as clearinghouses for information and contact points.

One of the major revolutions on the web in recent years has been the flurry of user-created content. This has manifested in widely known web sites such as YouTube, Facebook, and MySpace. Some public health outreach is already going on these sites. For example, Illumistream Health gives users access to a number of videos on various health topics targeted to teens and young adults (www.youtube.com/user/illumi stream). In self-defined communities like Yahoo Answers, users swap health tips and knowledge among themselves (under the Health tab at http://answers.yahoo.com). It should be noted that these sites can be and often are used to disseminate false and misleading information, ranging from AIDS conspiracy theories to false claims about the ineffectiveness of condoms for preventing the spread of STIs. Practitioners must be wary of using or directing others to these sites, even if reliable organizations upload information on them, because anyone can post on them and there is rarely any restriction or monitoring of the information posted.

Another useful intersection between information technology and health has been the rise of blogs, forums, and personal web sites devoted to specific ailments. These sites—though unregulated and frequently run by individuals who suffer from or know somebody who suffers from the ailment in question—can be an invaluable resource to those who want nonexpert opinions, a history of someone else's experience with the same issues, or just someone to commiserate with as they go through difficult times in their lives. These forums are an example of the Internet's ability to foster informal exchange of information and help create new communities sometimes linked through specific health issues. It is not necessarily clear how these communities can best be approached to improve potential outcomes at this juncture, but they merit attention.

A CHALLENGE AND AN OPPORTUNITY FOR PUBLIC HEALTH PRACTITIONERS

Public health practitioners' ability to take advantage of Web 2.0 will be crucial in shaping the future of public health initiatives in cyberspace. A typical Web 2.0 site will provide applications designed to help users publish their own content, including pictures, web journals (or blogs), profiles, and videos, and let the users create the content to share among themselves.

Some public health organizations targeting specific issues have already chosen to engage in these dynamic platforms by establishing their own accounts (the American Cancer Society, American Lung Association, and American Heart Association all have sites on Facebook, a popular Web 2.0 site as of this writing) or have attempted to utilize user-generated content for their traditional web sites (such as blogs or video recordings for the American Heart Association's Start Walking Campaign). As people spend more of their free time on and base more of their activities on these web sites, it will be important for public health practitioners to establish presences and links within them. Web 2.0 sites offer opportunities to target specific communities because people organize themselves geographically and by interest.

This organization will also allow a better interface between larger public health groups and community-specific resources. For example, the American Heart Association could target people in specific urban areas and recommend walking and biking trails to them, as well as resources for cheap cardiac screening and treatment of heart ailments. Or the American Cancer Society could target specific communities at higher risk for specific types of cancer and give them information about appropriate screening techniques. As the Internet helps carve the great pie of mass media into smaller and smaller slices, community-targeted health messages will become more and more necessary and cost-effective. Internet tracking software is already being used to target advertisements at people in specific groups (for example, dating sites often suggest available singles in the user's city), and similar technology can readily be used by community-specific services in a larger network to target individuals who may live in a specific geographic community or be members of another type of community.

Public health organizations can also use the Internet to reach out to communities that might not have the information resources they need to manage chronic disease. The Joslin Diabetes Center, for example, has experimented with a chat room that allows diabetes sufferers from around the world to communicate with one another, both for emotional support and for information-sharing purposes. By creating a virtual community focused on dealing with the symptoms, suffering, and requirements of living with diabetes, the chat room had a positive effect on most of its users (as measured by an e-mail survey) and offered a place where people from around the world could interact with others who shared a common trait (Zrebiac, 2005).

Blurring the Line Between Education and Entertainment

In future, information technology will affect community-based interventions in numerous and somewhat unpredictable ways. One thing that can be predicted with relative confidence is that many community-based interventions involving health education will be more interactive than at present. While it is critically important for public health practitioners to get information out into the communities where it is needed, it is equally important for the information to engage with members of those communities and for them to gain as much new knowledge as is possible. A web site that gets ignored or clicked through will be as useless as a pamphlet that sits untouched in a community center. Neither has the desired positive impact on the community's health.

As the Internet has evolved, many frequent surfers have become remarkably adept at seeking out the information they want. This skill can range from being able to target search inquiries to find specific information to the ability to scan a web page visually in such a way that advertising is never even seen. This sophistication will only increase in the future. While various technological fixes have been proposed and even implemented, such as ads that cover the entire screen to unskippable video, the easiest way to keep users from skipping the content is to make it a draw in and of itself. There are a number of ways to do this, but one that will likely prove fruitful in the future is the blurring of the boundaries between entertainment and education in the form of informative interactive experiences.

Using Computer Games to Reach a Community

One of the most reported on versions of the blurring of education and entertainment is Second Life, a virtual world in which hundreds of thousands of users spend significant amounts of time (and real money) socializing with one another. Second Life has been at the vanguard of a variety of Internet initiatives and has included everything from a virtual brothel to virtual campaign headquarters for real-life political campaigns. The American Cancer Society, again, has already established a presence in the world of Second Life, including executing a fund-raiser that garnered more than $100,000. It is clear that this virtual space, and others that will come in the future, have potential as places where public health practitioners and organizations can work at the virtual community level.

It is also worth asking whether people who are involved in such activities actually constitute new and evolving communities. For example, it has been suggested that gamers and heavy Internet users may have a higher incidence of certain ailments such as obesity and depression. Interventions targeting communities of people who are seriously involved in such activities and less likely to be reached through real-life activities might be quite effective.

Virtual Experience as an Intervention Method

Another potential use of emerging technologies is the creation of stand-alone games that allow people to directly experience some public health threat or means of intervention. An example of this phenomenon is the game series Pandemic, where the player takes on the role of a disease attempting to wipe out humankind. While this particular game is of marginal educational value, the idea of using interactive entertainment to provide a more experiential method of learning is clearly feasible, given sufficient funding and design. At the Food Force web site, sponsored by the United Nations World Food Program, users can download a game that simulates what it is like to try to feed a large population with extremely limited resources (www.food-force .com). The site also includes data on the actual World Food Program and the problems of hunger in the world today.

The World Food Program also runs a web site called Free Rice, where game players match vocabulary words and earn virtual grains of rice (www.freerice.com). Sponsors then pay to have an equal number of actual grains of rice sent to hungry communities around the world. Both games are entertaining, and both serve an important function in alerting players to the serious problem of hunger and providing a starting point for them to do their own research on the matter. There is no reason why this approach, if modified, would not work with other public health issues, such as managing chronic diseases or risky behaviors.

The space for continued investigation and experimentation in this area is as yet mostly untapped. This fact is especially important when you consider that many games glorify potentially dangerous behaviors. It has long been suggested that the smoking and heavy drinking portrayed in movies promote public health hazards that cause harm to many communities, and yet such behaviors are rampant in popular games. The Metal Gear Solid games feature tobacco use, while the popular Grand Theft Auto series contains, among other things, heavy alcohol and drug use, as well as implied sexual activity without protection. It is difficult to imagine that such imagery would have less influence than images on television or in movies, and it is well established that such games are frequently purchased for and played by minors. Providing alternatives to the community of young gamers that promote healthy lifestyles and choices would seem to be a good use of resources.

Using Cell Phones and Smartphones for Community Intervention

Computers and the Internet are not the only players on the technological landscape that may be important to community public health. Another very significant development is the expansion of cell phone networks and technology. Cell phones not only provide the same services as traditional wired phones but also frequently have additional features beyond portability. Text messages, for example, are a cheap and effective way of sending short messages instantaneously to individuals or groups. One example of the utility of this tool in interventions is the use of text alerts to remind people to take medication on schedule, encourage check-ins for various programs, or provide positive reinforcement for an ongoing effort like a smoking cessation program. A text message sent at specific times is a potentially affordable way to send effective reminders of information and reinforce messages. Two recent studies showed promising results in using cell phones to disseminate sex information and remind HIV-positive patients to take their medicine at the appropriate time via text messages (Ybarra & Bull, 2007). These sorts of interventions are very cost-effective and take advantage of an item that is becoming virtually a requirement of modern life. A pamphlet with crucial information about safe sex might be discarded or forgotten, but if that information is accessible via cell phone it will be available any time the user has access to his or her phone. For modern teens and young adults, the extent of this access might come close to twenty-four hours a day.

As cell phone technology improves, so will its potential uses in promoting community health. Apple's iPhone can already be used to read news and e-mail and has tools useful for issues like weight management (such as a pedometer application, calorie calculators, and restaurant locators that can suggest healthy choices in the area). Today's high-tech toy readily becomes tomorrow's standard-issue device, and as smartphones proliferate so will opportunities for interventions utilizing them.

Chat applications will allow sponsors to text in real time with addicts who need rein-forcement to avoid relapsing. Electronic databases of food information will allow peo-ple to make more informed choices about what they put into their bodies. Health and news alerts can be beamed directly to handsets, providing real-time updates about issues to people who are out of range of most news media.

Reaching Underserved Communities via New Communication Tools

Increased communication between health workers will allow for more efficient alloca-tion of resources and better awareness of what is going on from moment to moment. Translation services and dictionaries allow health workers to interface with members of communities with low levels of English fluency, even when linguistic needs are not anticipated. Electronic methods can also be used for data gathering. Surveys might be beamed through Bluetooth or another format to handsets and answered there at the user's leisure, potentially increasing response rates (while possibly also introducing other issues).

In communities previously underserved by communication technology, such as geographically isolated areas, communities with a high incidence of poverty or where transportation is difficult, cell phones offer the easiest and cheapest way to connect people to sources of information. Cell phones themselves could be used as tools of intervention in certain scenarios. A phone can be used to contact emergency services for help, advice, or information. Future technological advances may allow for addi-tional useful features. For example, high-definition photographs could be transmitted so that members of a virtual community could see other members as they engage in a group discussion or all participants could watch an intervention simultaneously before a discussion. Such advances are already underway, as people within the public health community are frequently invited to watch and participate in webinars.

A LIMITATION OF THE NEW TECHNOLOGIES

As new communication technologies become more and more commonplace, they will continue to integrate themselves into the lives of citizens and become useful as tools of public health and safety. It is important, then, for public health practitioners to be aware of both the accessibility of these technologies in specific communities and how widely they are used. While access to computers in the United States is nearly univer-sal at this point, thanks to libraries and community centers, such access cannot help people who do not know how to operate the computers. As more and more information and organizations go online and as more communication takes place there, it is essen-tial that awareness of the limits of technological access and technological literacy in any given community be a part of any public health initiative. Just as conventional illit-eracy can render even the most well thought out and informative materials worthless, so can technological illiteracy and lack of access make even the best thought out and carefully constructed web page, chat room, or podcast useless.

Steps like holding computer training programs at libraries to teach people how to go online and search for health information and encouraging children to print out materials at school and take them home to their parents can help ameliorate this issue and make materials exponentially more effective in communities where Internet access is still limited. One Chicago study showed that giving Internet access to citizen leaders in a neighborhood was effective in raising their feelings of empowerment, but less effective than anticipated in improving empowerment among neighbors and other members of the community (Masi, Suarez-Balcazar, Cassey, Kinney, & Plotrowski, 2003). Though the study was small in scope, its results may imply that for the Internet to be a truly egalitarian resource it must be available in every home. Another study showed that when disadvantaged girls as young as eight were given Internet access and access to a program designed to help them make healthy choices, they ate more fruits and vegetables and increased their levels of exercise (Thompson et al., 2008).

The Internet and associated technologies offer great promise as tools for combating the health issues that plague various communities, but it is important to make sure that as we move forward no one is left behind.

SUMMARY

In this chapter we have ventured beyond community as defined and limited by geography to explore how technology has enabled us to begin defining, developing, and reaching communities globally. While at present access is limited in many vulnerable populations, as technology continues to spread among youth and young adults, it will become a common tool for public health practitioners to use in the design of community-based interventions.

ACTIVITIES

1. Select a health problem and formulate a way to develop an online community-based intervention to address it.

2. Think of a new iPhone app (application) that could become a useful tool for a community-based intervention. (You may assume that everyone in this community has an iPhone.)

3. Pick a health problem and conduct a literature search to see how public health practitioners have used the Internet to address it.

4. As discussed in this chapter, communities are not defined solely by geographic boundaries. Identify two examples of nongeographic communities in which you are involved.

DISCUSSION QUESTIONS

1. How might gaming be used to teach practitioners to perform community-based health interventions?

2. What advantages are there in developing interventions for virtual communities who meet only in cyberspace?

3. Can you think of a recent technological development that has improved the health of the community you live in?

4. Discuss a recent technological development and how it could be used as a tool for intervention.

COMMUNITY-BASED HEALTH INTERVENTIONS IN PRACTICE

OVERVIEW

This chapter consists of a collection of case studies in which community-based health interventions have been undertaken in a variety of settings to address health problems such as arthritis, asthma, adult vaccinations, alcohol use, cardiovascular disease, childhood immunizations, injuries from motor vehicle accidents, sexual violence, and tobacco use. These examples are not intended as an exhaustive account of community-based interventions, but rather as insights into the numerous approaches public health practitioners are currently developing and applying. Each case study follows a broadly similar structure, beginning with a discussion of the health problem being addressed, proceeding to a look at the intervention employed and a summary of its evaluation, and concluding with questions to provoke further thoughts. An evaluation was carried out in most of these case studies, and when an evaluation is absent readers are asked to consider how they would design and implement an evaluation for the intervention. Furthermore, a reference citation has been provided for each case study to encourage and enable continued discussion about these interventions.

ARTHRITIS

Arthritis interferes with or limits sufferers' usual daily activities. In Minnesota over a quarter of adults have been diagnosed as having arthritis, and almost two-fifths of people age fifty-five and older experience limitations in their activities. While early diagnosis and treatment can diminish the disability associated with the disease, less than one percent of individuals who suffer from arthritis seek help. Treatment options routinely include physical activity and self-management education, and community-based interventions that provide these services to individuals with or at risk for arthritis can reduce both physical and financial burdens associated with the disease.

The Intervention

Sponsored by the Centers for Disease Control and Prevention (CDC), the Minnesota Arthritis Program employed a systems approach to link the state's elderly to arthritis intervention programs. It did this by developing partnerships between programs that have overlapping goals and serve the same target population. Specifically, the Minnesota Arthritis Program partnered with the Elderberry Institute's Living at Home Block Nurse program, a program that works to help the elderly remain in their homes. Through this partnership, arthritis-focused services that included self-management education were integrated with existing programs that offer independent living assistance. The program targeted people aged sixty-five and older who lived in Elderberry senior housing units to participate in the intervention. The program used both health professionals and neighborhood volunteers to provide health care and supportive services. The partnership enhanced the number of program participants and expanded its program leaders and exercise program instructors.

The Evaluation

Evaluation results indicated that progress was made in achieving the goal. Specifically, in 2006 there was a significant increase in self-help program leaders (from 21 to 67), and the number of arthritis exercise program instructors likewise increased (from 19 to 35). These increases led to a rise in the number of participants, from 98 to 308. The number of Minnesota's 87 counties with intervention programs also increased from 14 to 50, significantly improving access.

Your Further Thoughts

1. What type of evaluation do you believe was planned and carried out to determine program effectiveness? Make sure to name data measures and sources.

2. How would you evaluate this intervention to be certain that other factors did not improve the awareness of elderly people with arthritis about what they needed to do to remain healthy?

REFERENCE

CDC's National Center for Chronic Disease Prevention and Health Promotion. Minnesota: Evidence-based arthritis intervention programs among older adults across the state. Retrieved from www.cdc.gov/NCCDPHP/examples/index.htm.

ASTHMA

Asthma has reached epidemic levels, affecting nearly 20 million Americans, of which 6.3 million are children, making asthma the most common chronic disease among children (CDC, 2004a; CDC, 2004b). Consequently, asthma is the leading cause of school absenteeism, hospitalizations, emergency department visits, and deaths in children. The implications of persistent asthma-related problems reach far beyond the individual, imposing a mental and financial burden on family members who miss days of work to attend to asthma-related emergencies. While the condition is common across all races, children of color—especially Hispanic and African American children—are more likely on the national level to suffer from or die from asthma. The leading reasons for this disparity include poor asthma management knowledge, inadequate health care access, and indoor and outdoor air pollutants.

The Intervention

To decrease school absenteeism and hospitalization rates and help elementary school-aged youth manage their asthma, the American Lung Association (ALA) works to disseminate a proven effective school-based intervention program called Open Airways for Schools (OAS; see www.cdc.gov/asthma/interventions/openairway.htm). Originally designed and evaluated by Columbia University's College of Physicians and Surgeons, this program aims to increase children's ability to recognize their asthma symptoms, increase their capacity to manage their asthma, and enhance their ability to communicate with their parents about asthma.

This child-centered initiative is offered during the school day in six forty- to sixty-minute educational sessions conducted over the course of two to three weeks. OAS facilitators carry out the educational sessions after they are trained by ALA staff on basic asthma education, including the purpose and usage of different asthma medical equipment such as peak flow meters and inhalers. Overall the OAS educational program focuses on helping children gain control over their asthma. The topics covered in the curriculum include basic information about asthma, recognizing and managing asthma symptoms, using asthma medicines, identifying and controlling triggers, and handling problems related to asthma and school. Before being disseminated by the ALA, this program was evaluated by Evans and associates in 1987.

The Evaluation

Evans and colleagues (1987) employed an experimental research design to determine the program's effectiveness. Utilizing six pairs of middle schools (twelve schools total) in New York City that were matched by ethnic composition and size, the researchers randomly provided children in six of the schools the asthma education intervention. To recruit student participants, teachers sent letters home to parents in both English and Spanish. Eligibility criteria included being in the third, fourth, or fifth grade, parents reporting that the child had had at least three asthma episodes in the past year, and signed parental consent. The outcome measures used to evaluate changes in asthma knowledge, attitudes, beliefs, and skills in middle school children included self-management skills, self-efficacy, influence on parental decision making, school attendance and performance, children's attitudes, and parental report on the frequency, duration, and severity of their child's asthma episodes. In total the study comprised 239 students from 237 families ($n = 105$ for the control group; $n = 134$ for the intervention group). Data were collected a year following the intervention, and the researchers found that children who had been exposed to the intervention had increased their asthma management skills and self-efficacy and were influential in the decisions their parents made about their asthma. They had fewer self-reported asthma attacks, fewer symptom days, and indicated using more actions to manage their asthma compared with children in the control group.

Your Further Thoughts

1. How might this asthma education program be incorporated into the existing school curriculum without disrupting the school's schedule?

2. In what ways could parents' involvement in this program be expanded? How would you recruit parent participants?

3. Name possible process measurements that could be used for the evaluation of this program.

REFERENCES

Centers for Disease Control and Prevention. (2004a). Morbidity and Mortality Weekly Reports: Asthma prevalence and control characteristics by race/ethnicity—United States, 2002. Retrieved April 14, 2009, from www.cdc.gov/mmwr/preview/mmwrhtml/mm5307a1.htm.

Centers for Disease Control and Prevention. (2004b). Morbidity and Mortality Weekly Reports: Surveillance for asthma—United States, 1980–1999. Retrieved April 14, 2009, from www.cdc.gov/mmwr/preview/mmwrhtml/ss5101a1.htm.

Evans, D., Clark, N. M., Feldman, C. H., Rips, J. L., Kaplan, D. L., Levison, M. J., Wasilewski, Y., Levin, B., & Mellins, R. B. (1987). A school asthma health education program for children aged 8 to 11 years. *Health Education Quarterly, 14,* 267–279.

ADULT VACCINATIONS

Due to their success in lowering morbidity and mortality as well as decreasing medical costs, annual flu shots have been recommended for people living in the United States over the age of fifty, and for those of any age with chronic medical conditions. Nevertheless, a majority of hard-to-reach, high-risk populations such as undocumented immigrants, sex workers, substance users, and the homebound elderly fail to get vaccinated.

The Intervention

This intervention utilized a community-based participatory research (CBPR) methodology and was carried out in some underserved areas of New York City. Venue-Intensive Vaccines for Adults (VIVA)—a three-year project developed by a collaboration of groups including community residents, members of community-based organizations (CBOs), the local health department, and academic organizations—developed an intervention using CBPR to determine the challenges in reaching the groups defined as hard to reach, such as substance abusers and sex workers. The aim of VIVA was to "develop, implement and assess a rapid-vaccination protocol for hard-to-reach populations that would increase interest in vaccinations, provide free vaccinations during two flu seasons, and establish a model for the rapid vaccination of individuals that could be generalizable to other urban areas."

Neighborhoods that had an existing partnership with one of the VIVA CBOs were selected for the intervention. The project staff first conducted outreach using a variety of methods to estimate the size of the hard-to-reach populations in the selected neighborhoods and to gather surveys on the barriers to vaccination to develop the intervention strategy. Neighborhood outreach workers distributed fliers door-to-door about the project, comic strips on myths about vaccination, and the locations of free vaccine clinics. In January 2005, the selected neighborhoods were randomly assigned to either receive a pilot vaccination intervention (to evaluate the acceptance of vaccination) or to receive a rapid vaccination (a protocol developed for hard-to-reach populations). An outreach worker and a clinician were involved for eight weeks in both interventions, going door-to-door in apartment buildings offering vaccinations. Afterward the researchers conducted a survey to assess whether people living in the intervention areas were more interested in being vaccinated than people in areas without the intervention.

The Evaluation

In comparing interest in being vaccinated before and after the intervention among the hard-to-reach population, it was found that all people living in the intervention neighborhood, including the hard-to-reach population, were more interested in being vaccinated after the intervention than before. The authors concluded that using CBPR enabled them to gain the trust of the population that they were trying to reach. The authors also found that those who had been vaccinated previously were more receptive to being vaccinated again.

Your Further Thoughts

1. Do you think these findings can be generalized to other areas of the country? Why or why not?

2. What would be needed to sustain the interest of hard-to-reach populations in being vaccinated over time?

REFERENCE

Coady, M. H., Gates, S., Blaney, S., Ompad, D., Sisco, S., & Viahov, D. (2008). Project VIVA: A multilevel community-based intervention to increase influenza vaccination rates among hard-to-reach populations in NYC. *American Journal of Public Health, 98*(7), 1314–1321.

ALCOHOL USE

High rates of alcohol use among young adults result in a significant number of unintentional injuries. A variety of environmental strategies has been used to decrease the use of alcohol among adolescents, including enforcement of drinking and driving laws, policy changes in beverage sales, and reducing access to underage drinkers. The majority of these strategies have been implemented at the broader community level. To assess the effectiveness of neighborhood-level strategies that might be appropriate in situations with more limited resources, this program used an environmental approach to reduce young people's access to alcohol in two low-income communities.

The Intervention

Using a logic model to visually demonstrate the links between formal access to alcohol outlets, drinking, and alcohol-related problems, intervention activities focused on five different components over a five-year period: development of mobilization committees to provide direction; delivery of education presentations in a variety of languages, formats, and venues to reach various communities; targeting of education on responsible beverage service to outlets that sell or serve alcohol; and strengthening of enforcement efforts to prohibit alcohol sales to minors.

The Evaluation

In addition to monitoring sales to minors, researchers used outcome measures of police calls for assaults and public drunkenness, emergency medical services (EMS) calls for assaults and motor vehicle accidents, and EMS calls related to alcohol and other drugs. The results showed a one-third reduction in sales to minors and significant reductions in police and EMS calls for assaults and accidents.

Your Further Thoughts

1. How would implementing these intervention activities at the neighborhood level be more cost-effective than at the wider community level?

2. What community agencies or stakeholders would have to be mobilized in planning an intervention such as this?

3. The activities of this intervention took place over a five-year period. Would implementation of selected activities for a shorter period of time show a significant impact? Why or why not?

REFERENCE

Treno, A., Gruenewald, P., Lee, J., & Remer, L. (2007). The Sacramento Neighborhood Alcohol Prevention Project: Outcomes from a community prevention trial. *Journal of Studies on Alcohol and Drugs, 68,* 197–207.

CARDIOVASCULAR DISEASE

Currently, chronic diseases such as cardiovascular disease kill seven of every ten Americans each year. Many community-based interventions focus on preventing these diseases because these conditions can kill, disable (limiting people's ability to engage in daily life activities), and require costly medical care. By comparison, successful community-based interventions aimed at preventing chronic conditions are relatively inexpensive and have the potential to make a real difference in reducing morbidity and mortality.

In New York, practitioners sought through a community-based intervention known as the New York Healthy Hearts Program (NYHHP) to decrease morbidity associated with heart disease and stroke. In particular, this program employed a social marketing campaign to increase people's awareness of stroke signs and symptoms. The campaign was launched after Capital Region Stroke Task Force members found through targeted focus groups that residents of the Albany region of New York were aware of stroke symptoms, but were unaware of the need for rapid treatment for the symptoms of a stroke. In addition, they discovered that residents avoided calling for ambulance services because they feared having to pay out of pocket for the transport service if the symptoms were found to be unrelated to a stroke.

The Intervention

NYHHP implemented a multimedia awareness campaign targeting residents in the Albany region of the state. Using the acronym FAST (for face, arms, speech, and time) to indicate the symptoms of a stroke, the campaign urged people to dial 911 as quickly as possible after symptoms appear and informed them that pain was not necessarily involved with serious stroke symptoms. The intervention utilized a variety of media sources to deliver its messages. For example, NYHHP staff purchased radio and television time. After gaining some financial support from area hospitals, the program staff purchased space on buses and bus shelters for the display of informational materials. Members of the Stroke Task Force also made a number of presentations to community groups.

The Evaluation

Using pre- and posttest results, the evaluation compared the Albany region with a control region in New York that did not receive the multimedia campaign. Results revealed that Albany region residents were significantly more likely to report having viewed the television ads, and individuals who reported seeing the information were more likely to report that they would quickly call 911 if they or another appeared to be experiencing stroke symptoms.

In addition to knowledge, the evaluators examined behavior by collecting data from the area hospitals to determine how quickly residents got to the hospital after the onset of stroke symptoms. The results were encouraging, as a statistically significant number of stroke patients arrived at the hospital by ambulance.

Your Further Thoughts

1. Can you think of activities the researchers could have done other than using the media and speakers in the community?

2. What would you call this evaluation design?

3. How might the evaluation methodology be improved, and what additional information would be gained from this improvement?

REFERENCE

CDC's National Center for Chronic Disease Prevention and Health Promotion. New York: Heart disease and stroke—stroke awareness campaign. Retrieved from www.cdc.gov/NCCDPHP/examples/index.htm.

CHILDHOOD VACCINATIONS

In many communities infants and children do not receive immunizations at the recommended age. Children who are off schedule are susceptible to illnesses and deplete the community effect of **herd immunity.**

The Intervention

A curriculum was designed to teach pregnant women from public prenatal clinics in San Diego about the importance of infant immunization schedules and provide them with techniques they could use to keep their children's immunizations on schedule. During third-trimester prenatal visits, women in the intervention group received a one-on-one, interactive, immunization education session and viewed a fifteen-minute video emphasizing immunization timing and the diseases that are prevented through immunization. Using the woman's estimated due date, the perinatal health educator developed a personalized immunization reminder calendar, with the standard two-, four-, six-, twelve-, and fifteen-month schedule printed at the top, along with a reminder refrigerator magnet to hold the calendar in place. A comparison group of women received individual education and viewed a video on preventing sudden infant death syndrome (SIDS).

The Evaluation

At the start of both the intervention and comparison sessions, participants completed two questions about their knowledge of immunization schedules and infant sleep positions. The same questions were asked at the end of the sessions and in a telephone survey administered three months later. The county immunization registry was used to ascertain immunization status.

Of the 348 participants, 314 (90 percent) were able to be contacted at three months. Immunization knowledge increased significantly among women in the intervention group. There was no significant difference between the intervention and comparison group in the initiation of immunizations or the completeness of immunizations at ninety-two days (95 percent versus 93 percent).

Your Further Thoughts

1. Does it seem that a theoretical framework was used here? Why or why not?

2. What other outcome measures might have been used here?

3. How important is knowledge about immunization schedules to mothers bringing their children to visits where they receive immunizations?

REFERENCE

Uniag de Nuncio, M., Nader, P., Sawyer, M., De Guire, M., Prislin, R., & Elder, J. (2003). A prenatal intervention study to improve timeliness of immunization initiation in Latino infants. *Journal of Community Health, 28,* 151–165.

INJURIES FROM MOTOR VEHICLE ACCIDENTS

Children between the ages of eight and twelve are at increased risk for injuries from motor vehicle accidents, largely as a result of low rates of seat belt use and their front-seat position in cars.

The Intervention

In an Arkansas elementary school, researchers teamed up with school personnel to implement a variety of activities during the five-month intervention period. Using the logo Cubs Click It for Safety (styled after the school's tiger cub mascot), activities included education for staff, morning and afternoon announcements on the school's closed-circuit television, school assemblies, a highly visible bulletin board display, and poster distribution. A visual display and voice messages in the daily morning announcements contained an image buckling a seat belt around the school mascot and reminding students, "Remember—Cubs Click It for Safety." The afternoon announcements also had a verbal message to use seat belts along with a "clicker" sound. Parents were included through educational brochures sent home throughout the school year and through safety themes at school picnics and the school's annual festival. During survey and observational data collection, additional educational materials were provided as well as wristbands when passengers and drivers were correctly using seat belts and positions.

The Evaluation

Written and observational surveys about seat belt use and passenger positions were conducted before, during, and after the intervention activities. Students assisted in the collection of observational data. Campaign exposure was high, with 77 percent of parents and 89 percent of students having recall of campaign messages. Knowledge about restraint use and positioning increased among both parents and students. Restraint use by students increased from 71 percent to 91 percent ($p < .001$).

Your Further Thoughts

1. While the authors give equal weight to the findings of improvement in both knowledge and behavior, which would you consider to be a more significant indication of intervention success? Why?

2. At what ecological level did this intervention occur? Around what level of prevention were activities focused?

3. Would such an intervention be possible for a student to conduct? Why or why not?

REFERENCE

Aitken, M., Mullins, S., Lancaster, V., & Miller, B. (2007). "Cubs Click It for Safety": A school-based intervention for tween passenger safety. *Journal of Trauma, Injury, Infection, and Critical Care, 63,* S39–S43.

SEXUAL ASSAULT AND RELATIONSHIP VIOLENCE

Sexual violence against women is a national problem that occurs frequently on college and university campuses. One in four women will experience some form of sexual violence in her lifetime, whether in the form of relationship violence, rape, or stalking. Strong evidence suggests that sexual violence reporting rates on campuses are low, whether because of cultural acceptance, lack of knowledge about resources, or embarrassment.

The Intervention

Using an ecological framework, a universitywide series of activities was implemented to prevent sexual assault and relationship violence. The researchers suggest that this "case study of process" serve as a model for how a prevention program might be implemented by others in a similar setting. The planning process began with the development of a broad universitywide task force that included stakeholders from campus groups throughout the university. The task force's primary responsibilities were creating a vision for and suggesting how the institution would respond to sexual assault and relationship violence. To these ends, task force representatives were required to conduct environmental scans and a needs assessment to understand the campus climate, infrastructure, and resources for prevention. Current practices were compared to community benchmarks. This information was used to make and prioritize recommendations and suggestions on how to address needs.

The Evaluation

No impact evaluation activities were discussed.

Your Further Thoughts

1. What resources would be necessary to implement a similar process on your college campus?

2. What would be a reasonable timeline for implementation of this process on a college campus?

3. What type of evaluation might be used to assess the intervention?

REFERENCE

Lichty, L., Campbell, R., & Schuiteman, J. (2008). Developing a university-wide institutional response to sexual assault and relationship violence. *Journal of Prevention and Intervention in the Community, 36,* 5–22.

SMOKING

Cigarette smoking costs the United States an estimated $193 billion in tobacco-attributed health care expenditures and productivity loss and is responsible for approximately 438,000 premature deaths each year (CDC, 2008). In the United States, an estimated 20.8 percent of adults smoke cigarettes, and a substantial portion of these individuals are from age eighteen to twenty-four or twenty-five to forty-four (23.9 percent and 23.5 percent, respectively). To reduce smoking rates in these age groups, practitioners have targeted work sites, because nearly 63 percent of the adult population spends a third of each day at work (Moher, Hey, & Lancaster, 2003). Similarly, practitioners have begun to employ the Internet to implement smoking education and cessation interventions in work settings, as many employed adults use this technology on a daily basis.

The Intervention

Using work sites and an online intervention format, a smoking cessation program called Quit-Net® was implemented as part of a comprehensive health initiative to reduce smoking prevalence among International Business Machines (IBM) employees. To recruit participants, program announcements were sent to employees' intranet and e-mail accounts. To encourage participation, financial incentives in the form of insurance premium discounts were offered. During program enrollment, individuals were asked to self-report their smoking status. In total, 6,235 geographically dispersed self-identified smokers participated in IBM's health initiative. Of these, 1,713 IBM employees registered to use Quit-Net, a commercial web site offering tobacco cessation treatment consistent with national guidelines. Quit-Net subscriptions were paid for by IBM. When participants registered to use the Quit-Net web site, baseline data were collected. These included demographic information and smoking history, including current smoking rate, stage of change, number of twenty-four-hour quits in the past year, previous use of cessation treatments, and nicotine dependence. Once participants were registered, their web site utilization patterns were captured, and these data were recorded and included in the final analysis. Participants were followed for a twelve-month period.

The web site provided participants with online advice on how to quit smoking, aid in setting a quit date, assessment on motivation and nicotine dependence, tailored information on smoking risks, counseling aimed at building self-assessment skills, tailored assistance on choosing and using smoking cessation pharmacotherapies, and social support. These features were augmented with access to online cessation counselors, additional expert systems, and unlimited web-based social support.

The Evaluation

At twelve months postregistration, participants were asked to complete an online survey that assessed seven-day point-prevalence abstinence, actual quit date, number of twenty-four-hour quit attempts, longest duration of continuous abstinence, and use of cessation methods, including pharmacotherapies. Individuals who continued to smoke were asked to indicate their smoking rate, motivation for quitting, desire and confidence to quit, and time to first cigarette after waking. Of the 1,522 individuals who were surveyed at twelve-month follow-up, only 482 responded, resulting in a 32 percent response rate. The results showed a modest quit rate overall. Compared to those who used the site less frequently, those who used it four or more times during the twelve-month period were more likely to abstain from smoking. In addition, spending a greater amount of time on the site increased the likelihood of abstaining from smoking at twelve months. Also, those who used the augmented features such as online counseling were more likely to abstain from smoking compared to those who did not. The authors acknowledge a number of intervention limitations, including the facts that a low response rate limits the finding's generalizability and lack of a comparison group makes it difficult to determine whether employees would have abstained from smoking in the absence of the intervention.

Your Further Thoughts

1. Even though this intervention had only modest results, briefly state the steps you would take in planning this program for a smaller work site. Which approaches would you keep and which would you change? Why?

2. Survey response is critical, as it provides the data that will be needed to evaluate a program. Briefly describe steps that would increase the response rate.

3. Name possible process measurements that could be used for evaluation.

REFERENCES

Centers for Disease Control and Prevention. (2008). *Preventing tobacco use.* Retrieved August 31, 2009, from www.cdc.gov/nccdphp/publications/factsheets/Prevention/pdf/tobacco.pdf.

Graham, A. L., Cobb, N. K., Raymond, L., Sill, S., & Young, J. (2007). Effectiveness of an Internet-based worksite smoking cessation intervention at 12 months. *Journal of Occupational and Environmental Medicine, 49*(8), 821–828.

Moher, M., Hey, K., & Lancaster, T. (2003). Workplace interventions for smoking cessation. *Oxford Update Software, 3,* 1–59.

SUMMARY

The aim of this chapter was to highlight the wide variety of approaches currently being used by public health practitioners to address public health issues. It is evident that practitioners work in different settings—from schools to work sites to neighborhoods—in an effort to reach and improve the health of their target population. In some cases, though, evaluations were not carried out despite their being highly encouraged in the field of public health. This is a particular issue in relation to funding because in the absence of evaluation data that specifies program effectiveness, it is difficult to demonstrate the need for further funding or for program replication. We hope this chapter will encourage discussion of past interventions and that from these insights lessons for future practice will emerge.

GLOSSARY

Abstract   The summary of a research paper commonly found at the beginning of the document.

Active consent   The signing of a consent form by a parent or legal guardian of a child research subject allowing the child's participation in a research study.

Activities   The specific actions carried out as part of an intervention.

Activities approach model   A model that focuses on the activities of the project and its expected results and helps determine the resources needed to carry out the activities.

Advocacy coalition framework   A conceptual model that outlines processes involved in implementing policy-level social change.

Alma Ata Declaration   A 1978 World Health Organization policy stating that all individuals should have access to adequate and affordable primary health care and emphasizing the importance of involving communities in the delivery of primary health care.

Anonymity   A method of protecting the privacy of research participants by not collecting identifying information such as names, making it almost impossible to connect participants to their responses.

Assumptions   Unspoken understandings or conclusions about a research population's beliefs or behaviors made without any confirming data.

Attrition   The loss of participants in an intervention because they dropped out, were lost to follow-up, or died.

Background and significance   The section of a research paper or proposal that provides an overview of the problem, prior research related to the problem, and gaps in this research as justification for the proposed intervention.

Baseline data   The initial information collected about intervention participants that can be used as a comparison for data collected after an intervention has been implemented.

Basic priority rating system   A system for developing priorities in public health activities when resources are limited. The use of a variety of data sources allows for quantification of disease problems or risk factors by prevalence, cost, and severity.

Behavioral capability   A construct of social cognitive theory suggesting that an individual's knowledge about and skills related to a particular behavior affect the performance of that behavior.

Behavioral change theory   One of several theories that provide a systematic framework for understanding how and why individuals change their behavior.

Blogs   Posts by authors, usually on a single topic, that may range from public policy to entertainment to child rearing to an author's personal life. Many blogs are maintained by single authors, but some have several. Many use extensive hyperlinking, and some include videos.

Bluetooth   A wireless networking technology facilitating data transmission and device interfacing over short distances.

Boilerplate information   Text in a funding proposal indicating the facilities and support available at an institution. Generally included are a brief description of the institution's goals, mission, history, and resources, such as computer facilities and library.

Boolean operators   Logic statements that focus or connect main terms in database searches (such as *AND, OR,* and *NOT*).

Budget   A plan detailing and explaining the expenses that will be incurred as a result of an intervention and evaluation.

Budget justification   Statements that describe the need for each of the items and the precise roles of each staff member that have been listed in the budget of the intervention and evaluation.

Capacity assessment   An evaluation of the ability of a community or organization to effectively plan and implement an intervention.

Case finding   A strategy used to identify and reach out to high-risk individuals who are most affected by a specific health problem and/or least likely to perform a behavior that will improve their health.

Change theories   Theories that explain how organizations change over time.

CINAHL (Cumulative Index to Nursing and Allied Health Literature)   An electronic database that indexes literature relevant to community health from 1937 to the present.

Closed-ended question   A type of question used in research instruments to collect data that forces respondents to select an answer among the list of categories offered or provide a one-word response (such as a number, or yes or no).

Cochrane Review   An online resource that describes interventions on many topics and reviews the evidence on the strengths of the initiatives (www.cochrane.org/reviews).

Code of ethics   A guide to the everyday conduct of professionals in a specific field that holds them accountable for their actions. In public health, this code provides a standard for working in community settings and conducting research.

Community   A group of people connected by visible and invisible links and defined by geographic, physical, or political boundaries (geographic community) or by a shared interest, behavior, risk, or characteristic (communities of interest, such as racial, ethnic, or national background, and social units such as age, occupational status, or disease status).

Community advisory board   A formal group of stakeholders from the community who can provide input during the assessment or evaluation phase of an intervention.

Community assessment   A systematic review of a community's strengths and weaknesses relevant to health.

Community-based health intervention   An intervention designed to address a specific health need in a community by preventing or changing nonmedical factors that affect health.

Community-based participatory research (CBPR)   A type of research in which members and stakeholders in the targeted communities are actively involved in all stages of the research process.

Community Guide   A CDC-sponsored online resource that reviews and makes recommendations on evidence-based programs on a large variety of health topics (www.thecommunityguide.org).

Community input   Primary data collected from community members, service providers, and others who are knowledgeable about the health needs and health concerns of a community.

Community level   One of the levels of influence on health behavior in an ecological model. Interventions at this level work to change environmental or social structures.

Community setting   The environment or geographical area in which a community is located.

Concepts   The individual components or building blocks of a theory.

Confidentiality   A method of protecting the rights of research participants through procedures ensuring that no identifying information will be revealed to anyone other than the research team.

Consent form   A written document informing participants of the specific details of the study, such as the purpose, expectations, and the risks and benefits of participating in the research.

Constructs   Conceptual or schematic ideas that are grouped to form a theory.

Control group   The unit of analysis that does not receive the treatment or intervention and serves as a comparison group for statistical purposes.

Convenience sample   A type of sample that is obtained by nonrandomly enrolling participants who are available at the time of the project.

Cross-tabulation   A type of analysis that examines the distribution of at least two variables at the same time and usually presents them in a table.

Cyberspace   A metaphor for the content and interaction on the Internet and other computer networks.

Data   A collection of pieces of information that help increase knowledge about a topic of interest.

Data processing   The conversion of raw data into a form that can be processed by computer and manipulated into variables for analysis.

Data set   A collection of variables related to a specific topic, typically organized with a computer software program.

Demographic variables   The personal characteristics of individuals or populations (such as age, education, occupation, and race) that can describe both geographic and common-interest communities.

Descriptive analysis   A type of statistical analysis that summarizes the characteristics of a sample and examines how variables relate to one another.

Discussion guide   A manual used during focus group meetings consisting of a set of questions developed prior to the discussion.

Dose   The amount or strength of an intervention delivered to the target population; can be measured in time (days, weeks, months, or years) and/or in terms of the number of practitioners delivering the intervention to the target population.

Ecological level   The perspective from which you analyze the network of organizations or individuals in the social environment.

Ecological theory   A theory emphasizing that health is the result of a dynamic interplay of individual-level characteristics with the physical and social environment. Individuals, families, and communities are not isolated entities, but rather an interrelated ecological system with each adapting to changes occurring in other parts of the organization.

Economic asset   A type of physical or commercial resource that can positively address the health needs of a community.

EMBASE   A biomedical electronic database covering literature on a wide variety of health and medical topics, including health policy and management, public health, occupational health, and environmental health.

Ethical conduct   The carrying out of an intervention in a way that treats participants with respect and causes no harm to them or the community (*see* Code of ethics).

Evaluation   A systematic assessment of the effectiveness of an intervention, program, or policy. Evaluations not only assess the outcome of the intervention, but also determine whether the objectives of an intervention were met, how the components were implemented, and the extent to which these components contributed to achieving the objectives.

Expectations   A construct of social cognitive theory positing that individual perceptions of the probability of a desired outcome affect the performance of the behavior leading to the outcome.

Experimental group   The unit of analysis that receives the intervention or treatment of interest.

Facebook   A social networking site on the Internet (*also see* MySpace).

Facilitator   An individual who leads or conducts a focus group and makes sure that all questions of interest are answered and all members of the group share their input (also known as a moderator).

Facilitators   Items such as travel funds to cover participants' travel expenses that help research investigators recruit participants.

Fidelity   The degree to which an adapted or tailored existing intervention is true to the original design, content, and implementation plan.

Fiscal agent   An organization or institution that receives and monitors grant funding for another agency or group.

Five Ps   A marketing strategy for guiding the design of social marketing campaigns that uses the concepts of product, price, place, promotion, and positioning.

Focus group   A method of data collection in qualitative research where small groups of six to twelve participants are brought together to share their opinions and views about a defined topic. The group discussion is facilitated by a moderator who is part of the research team.

Follow-up question   A technique used in research to clarify or obtain additional information following a response to a preceding question.

Forced-choice question   A type of question used in research instruments that has limited choice responses; the wording of the question requires the respondent to provide a specific response (such as agree or disagree, or true or false).

Fringe benefits   Mandated expenses such as Social Security, worker's compensation insurance, and state unemployment insurance and voluntary benefits (such as health insurance and retirement programs) that are expressed as a percentage of personnel salaries.

Gamers   People who play computer games.

Gantt chart   A visual timeline in units of weeks, months, or years detailing the anticipated start and stop dates of planned evaluation and activities

Global Health Database   An electronic database that provides access to research related to communicable diseases, tropical diseases, parasitic diseases, human nutrition, community and public health, and medicinal and poisonous plants from an international perspective.

Google Scholar   The academic arm of the Google web site.

Group interviews   Questions and discussion about a topic with two or more people.

Group level   One of the levels of influence on health behavior and outcomes in the ecological perspective. Intervention at this level works to change knowledge, attitudes, and practices about a health issue among members of a target group.

Herd immunity   The overall protective effect that ensues when a majority of community members are immune to a disease by virtue of immunization or prior infection; those few who lack the immunity are very unlikely to come into contact with an infected person, thus preventing the occurrence of a chain of infection.

IDUs   Injecting drug users.

Impact evaluation   An assessment of the effects of an intervention and whether its objectives have been accomplished.

Incentives Small sums of money or gifts that are given to individuals for participating in an intervention, either as compensation for time or as a strategy for retention.

Individual resources Assets in the community of interest that positively address health needs, including individuals who have specific skills, are experienced in community-based work, or have the willingness to help improve the health of the community.

Individual rights The rights for freedom of actions granted by a government to individuals as opposed to civil or legal rights.

Informed consent A research subject's agreement to participate in a study based on a clear understanding of the nature of the study and what the individual will be asked to do.

In-kind contribution Nonfinancial resources, such as meeting facilities or staff time, that help support an intervention.

Inputs The resources, contributions, and investments that are needed to carry out the activities of an intervention.

Institutional resources Assets in the community of interest that can help address the health needs of the community, such as clinics, libraries, and recreational facilities.

Institutional review board (IRB) A formal committee established by an institution to review the ethics of all research projects involving human subjects being proposed by practitioners who work in that institution; works to ensure that the rights and welfare of research participants are protected.

Instruments The questionnaires, interview schedules, and research protocols used in a research project.

Internal validity The idea that any effects observed following an intervention were caused by the intervention.

Internet survey A questionnaire or survey administered through the Internet.

Key informants Individuals in the community who occupy leadership roles and can provide insight into the needs of the target population, their reaction to a particular intervention, and the impact of the intervention on the community.

Key stakeholders Community insiders—decision makers within service provision agencies, advisory boards, and leaders of community-based organizations who have a vested interest in the success of the community assessment or intervention.

Large data sets Secondary data sets available for analysis from other sources, such as national health web sites, health departments, universities, and research centers (*see also* Secondary data).

Letter of collaboration A statement to a funding agency written by a research team's collaborating agency describing its role and contribution to the study.

Letter of intent A written statement to a funding agency expressing the intention to apply for funding.

Levels of prevention The three main types of health promotion activities corresponding to the prevention, detection, and treatment of disease (*see also* Primary prevention, Secondary prevention, and Tertiary prevention).

Likert-type response A response format consisting of four to five options increasing or decreasing in magnitude (for example, strongly agree to strongly disagree, or vice versa).

Locator form A form containing the participant's basic and alternate contact information.

Logic model A way of describing the connection between various components in an intervention or program. Such descriptions are frequently put in the form of a diagram.

Mapping A technique in which two or more data elements are integrated or linked geographically using a computer software program specifically designed for this purpose.

Methods or **methodology** A set of scientific techniques used to systematically conduct research investigations such as intervention studies.

Minnesota Heart Health Project   One of the earliest community-based health interventions, implemented in 1980 and lasting approximately six years, aiming to lower the incidence of heart disease and stroke.

Moderator   The person who conducts and leads the discussion in a focus group (*also see* Facilitator).

Multilevel and structural equation modeling   A type of statistical manipulation in quantitative research in the behavioral sciences in which latent variables or random effects are introduced to explain correlations in responses.

MySpace   A social networking site on the Internet (*also see* Facebook).

National Guideline Clearinghouse   An online database initiated by the Agency for Healthcare Research and Quality (AHRQ) that provides access to evidence-based clinical practice guidelines.

Needs assessment   An approach to community assessment used to identify the needs, problems, and deficiencies of a particular community.

Networking   The act of linking to or making connections with people who have personal and professional experience in a particular public health area of interest.

Nominal group technique   A strategy for group decision-making in which the opinions of all members are taken into account; while several variations exist, one simple method is for members to each give a brief reason for their choice on an issue and order their preferences among the different options (that is, 1st, 2nd, 3rd, and so on); the option that the most members have indicated as their first choice is then selected.

North Karelia Project   An early community-based health intervention (1971) responding to community concern about the high mortality rate from heart disease in a predominantly rural area in Finland.

Objectives   Quantitative descriptions of what an intervention's activities will accomplish; usually they specify who is targeted by the intervention, what the intervention expects to change and by how much, and in what time frame.

Observational data   Data collected by the observer carefully noting the details of what is seen to transpire over a specific period of time or during an occasion.

Observational learning   A construct of social cognitive theory positing that exposure to the performance of an action or behavior by influential others can affect whether an individual engages in that action or behavior.

One-on-one face-to-face interview   A data collection technique in which the researcher poses questions to the respondent in person.

Open-ended question   A type of question used in research instruments to collect data that does not force participants to choose from a predetermined set of possible responses, but rather allows them to provide their own response.

Operationalize   The process of specifying how a particular construct or concept will be measured.

Organizational capacity   An organization's ability to successfully deliver its products or services, achieve its goals, and carry out its mission.

Organizational level   One of the levels of influence on health behavior in an ecological model that uses the shared connection between individuals to build changes in health behaviors and the environment.

Other expenses   An expense category in the budget that includes all miscellaneous costs that do not fit in the personnel or other than personnel services categories, such as postage, advertising, or subscriptions.

Other than personnel services (OTPS)   A budget category in a funding application that includes all non-personnel-related expenses, such as equipment, office supplies, and items necessary for the intervention.

Outcome approach model   An approach to constructing logic models that focuses on intended outcomes and how program components will be evaluated to determine whether they are achieving the intended results.

Outcome evaluation   A type of evaluation conducted at the end of an intervention study to determine whether the overall aims or goals were attained and can be attributed to the intervention rather than to other factors occurring around the same time; also assesses any unintended outcomes and weighs the costs and benefits of the intervention.

Outcome indicators   Variables used to measure the intended effects or success of the intervention on the targeted population.

Outcomes   The intended effects of the intervention on the targeted population.

Outliers   A value that is markedly different from other values in a data set.

Outputs   The specific components of the intervention, such as the activities and the targeted population.

Overall goal   The overarching aim of an intervention, corresponding to the health problem the intervention hopes to address; states the health problem in broad terms, how the intervention will address the health problem, and specifies the targeted population.

Parental consent   The permission of parents or guardians for the participation of children in a research study.

Participant observation   A field research data collection technique in which the researcher studies the phenomena of interest by sharing in the activities associated with it.

Partnerships   Alliances or collaborations that occur between researchers and individuals and groups in a community to aid in conducting community assessments, assessing priorities for action, developing community interventions, and evaluating outcomes.

Passive consent   A consent process typically used in school settings in which a document is sent home with the potential child research subject to inform the legal guardian about the study. If the legal guardian does not sign and return the form stating that the parent does *not* want the student to participate, the investigator assumes that the legal guardian has given the child permission to participate in the study.

PATCH (Planned Approach to Community Health)   Developed by the CDC, this is a five-phase planning model that aims to enhance community partnerships and link community participation with community-level epidemiology. PATCH's five phases are mobilizing the community, collecting and organizing data, choosing health priorities, developing a comprehensive intervention plan, and evaluation.

Pawtucket Heart Health Project   One of the early community-based health interventions, implemented in 1983 and lasting approximately eight years, to reduce stroke and cardiovascular disease rates. The community was mobilized through programs based at work sites, churches, nonprofit agencies, and social service programs.

Personnel   An expense category in the budget that includes all staff members' salaries and benefits; specifies how many individuals will be hired, their job titles, and the number of hours they will be working.

Physical structures   A type of resource or asset identified in a capacity assessment that refers to land, buildings, transportation, established infrastructure, and natural resources that could positively contribute to improving the health status of the community.

Pilot study   The initial testing of an intervention with the purpose of obtaining valuable feedback to improve the study before implementing it with the full population.

Placebo   A fake pill or noneffective treatment distributed, for example, to the comparison group in a randomized control trial.

Policy level   One of the levels of influence on health behavior and outcomes in the ecological perspective. Interventions at this level change laws or policies that will facilitate health (such as smoking bans and seat belt laws).

Population-based approach   An approach to addressing health behaviors based on the idea that risk behaviors are differentially distributed across a population and that small improvements in risk behaviors can yield significant results in health outcomes.

Power analysis   Power analysis is based on whether the study sample size can adequately detect changes through statistical analysis.

Pre- and post-survey   A research design in which baseline data is gathered at the very beginning of an intervention and again at the end of the intervention.

Precoding   The unobtrusive placement of data entry codes on a survey form, which facilitates inputting the information into a statistical computer program.

Preexisting data   *See* Secondary data.

Pre-post design   A type of quasi-experimental study design in intervention research in which the same survey is administered to program recipients before and after the intervention to examine changes in knowledge, attitude or behavior and other individual characteristics.

Primary data   Information that is collected firsthand and has not been analyzed previously.

Primary prevention   A level of prevention that aims to prevent a disease or condition before it begins.

Prioritize   A decision-making process used to categorize findings from community health needs assessments by level of urgency, ranging from the most to the least pressing issue.

Probe   A verbal technique used in qualitative research to elicit additional information from respondents relevant to addressing the research aim and/or research questions.

Problem statement   A statement explaining the problem that the intervention will address; includes who is being affected, where the problem is occurring, when it is occurring, and how the problem can and needs to be solved.

Process evaluation   A type of evaluation designed to assess how an intervention is being implemented, what aspects are working as planned or might need to be revised to reach the project's aims.

Process indicators   Variables used to assess how an intervention is being implemented and which aspects are working as planned or might need to be revised to reach the intended goal.

Program planning   The process of designing a community-based intervention.

Prospective cohort design   A research design in which subjects sharing a particular exposure (such as smoking or mammography screening) are followed over time to compare the occurrence of a particular health outcome (such as lung or breast cancer) between two groups.

Protection of human subjects   The ethical treatment of research participants; a core responsibility of public health researchers.

Psychometric properties   Analyses run on an instrument that demonstrate their validity and reliability.

Psychometrics   The measurement properties of a research instrument.

Public Health Partners   An online resource that provides access to public health journals, newsletters, and reports from government and community agencies (http://phpartners.org/guide.html).

PubMed   The National Library of Medicine's electronic archive of biomedical journals, which provides bibliographic, abstract, and full-text coverage of literature related to health management, health policy, and public health.

Qualitative data   An investigative methodology that emphasizes the quality of meaning through open-ended questions and observation.

Quantitative data   Research involving collection and analysis of data that can be expressed in numerical form.

Quasi-experimental design   A research design that incorporates some elements of a randomized-controlled trial or "true" experiment, but lacks the element of randomization to a treatment or control group.

Questionnaire   A research tool used to gather information from respondents.

Randomization   A procedure in which the unit of analysis is systematically selected into the study.

Randomized-controlled trial   A research study design in which subjects are randomly assigned to either a treatment or control group; often referred to as a "true" experiment.

Random sample   A type of sample in which the units of analysis have an equal probability of being selected into the study.

Rapid assessment procedure   Involves the tailoring of specific procedures and techniques for use in different cultural and geographic settings for programmatic purposes by people who may not necessarily possess high-level academic skills.

Reach   The ability of an intervention to access the target population.

Reciprocal determinism   A construct of social cognitive theory that emphasizes the bidirectional nature of interactions between individuals and their surrounding environment; that is, the environment influences individuals' behavior, but the actions of individuals also shape the environment.

Recruitment plan   A strategic plan for the goals of recruitment of participants into an intervention and how and when these goals will be met.

Reinforcement   A construct of social cognitive theory positing that responses (physical, mental, or verbal) to a particular behavior will affect whether the individual performs that behavior.

Reliability   The ability of an instrument or set of items to consistently measure the same construct each time it is used.

Request for applications (RFAs)   An announcement by a funding agency to solicit applications for funding, generally on a specific topic; synonymous with *Request for proposals.*

Request for proposals (RFPs)   An announcement by a funding agency to solicit proposals for funding, generally on a specific topic; synonymous with *Request for applications.*

Research utilization   The translation and implementation of research findings into actual practice.

Respondent fatigue   Overburdening a respondent with too many questions; the point at which a participant finds the number of questions on a survey to be excessive.

Risk behaviors   Negative health behaviors that increase the risk of disease, such as smoking, poor diet, or lack of physical activity.

Sample   A selection or part of the population for which data are collected and analyzed.

Sample size   The number of participants on which data analyses are based.

Saturation   The point in the collection of qualitative data at which no new information is being collected from additional respondents or the information being gathered becomes repetitive.

Scale   A group of questions that measure a specific construct or idea.

Scientific literature   Professional journals whose articles are the result of a peer review process.

Secondary data   Data collected from preexisting or precollected sets of information that can provide epidemiological clues to who is at risk, where people are at risk, and changes or trends over time in the distribution of the disease; a body of literature containing previously published articles on original research, commentaries, and reviews.

Secondary prevention   A level of disease prevention that focuses on screening and early diagnosis of a disease or condition.

Second Life   A "massively multiplayer" Internet game and interaction application created by Linden Labs.

Secular trends   Events that occur in the larger society that are unrelated to the intervention, such as medical improvements in diagnostic tools that may unintentionally affect health outcomes among participants.

Self-efficacy   A construct of social cognitive theory positing that an individual's belief in his or her ability to carry out a particular action will affect the performance of the action.

Semistructured interviews   A qualitative research or evaluation method in which participants are asked to respond to a series of open-ended questions.

SMART objectives   An acronym describing how objectives should ideally be written: specific, measurable, achievable, relevant, and time-bound.

Smartphones   Cell phones with a range of capabilities in addition to basic phone function, such as surfing the Internet, running computerlike applications, or accessing various kinds of information.

SMS (Short Message Service) text messages   Written messages of 160 characters or fewer transmitted to cell phones from other cell phones or Internet applications.

Snowball sample   A type of sample obtained by asking participants to refer other potential participants from their larger network.

Social cognitive theory   A learning and behavior change theory developed from social learning theory positing that people learn by observing the behaviors of others and that such learning occurs on both a cognitive and social level.

Social learning theory   A behavioral change theory suggesting that people learn through reinforcement, punishment, and observation of others.

Social marketing   The systematic application of marketing theory, strategies, and techniques to achieve a social goal such as smoking cessation or physical activity in a target population.

Specific aims   The initial section of most grant proposals that provides a succinct description of why, what, and how activities will be pursued; contains concrete objectives indicating how much change is expected as a result of the intervention over what time period and in which population.

Stage theory of organizational change   A framework for understanding how and why organizations initiate, implement, and evaluate new programs.

Stakeholders   Any person, group or organization that might be interested in or affected by the topic of a potential intervention.

Stanford Five-City Project   A longer, more comprehensive intervention than the earlier Stanford Three-City Project; implemented from 1980 to 1986 to change health behaviors that increase the risk of heart disease; included a more sophisticated mass media campaign.

Stanford Three-Community Study   An early community-based health intervention implemented in 1972 to test a communitywide intervention to change health behaviors that put residents at risk for cardiovascular disease; involved a mass-media campaign and group and individual education for high-risk individuals.

Statistical significance   The likelihood that a finding is true and not the result of chance.

Structural equation modeling   A sophisticated statistical analysis that can be conducted to demonstrate an intervention's impact at a variety of levels—for example, for an intervention conducted in several elementary schools, data can be analyzed on students in each class, the parents of the students, between classes, and between schools.

Structured interview guide   An interviewing guide used in qualitative research containing a series of predetermined questions to which the interviewer will return as the discussion proceeds and when respondents wander off topic.

Surfers   Internet users.

Sustainability   The ability of an intervention to continue beyond its period of initial funding.

Target community   The population, specific group of individuals, or community in which an assessment or intervention is focused.

Telephone surveys   A data collection method in which participants are contacted by telephone, usually through random selection of telephone numbers.

Tertiary prevention   A level of disease prevention that includes efforts to prevent disease progression after a risk factor or disease has been identified.

Theoretical frameworks   A suggested structure for how data fit together to explain or predict a dependent outcome; an organized way to think about behavior change and view the set of relationships between a health problem, target population, and program components and results.

Theory   An organized way to understand, explain, or predict relationships, behaviors, or outcomes.

Theory approach model   An approach to constructing logic models that uses theory to guide the planning and design of the intervention.

Timeline   A proposed schedule and systematic way of organizing an intervention or funding period by specifying the timing and activities that need to be accomplished.

Triangulation   The collection, analysis, and synthesis of data from a variety of sources and methods to obtain a greater depth of understanding; generally refers to the use of both quantitative and qualitative data.

Tuskegee Study   A research study conducted by the Public Health Service from 1932 to 1972 that investigated the natural history of syphilis in poor and illiterate African American men. Men were not informed about the actual purpose of the study, and even after the discovery of penicillin as an effective treatment for syphilis the men were not informed or treated for the disease. The deception involved in this study helped set the stage for establishing a code of ethics in the United States by which all researchers must abide. *See also* Code of ethics.

Two-group design   A research or evaluation method in which a second group that is roughly equivalent to the studied group is included in the design and analysis for comparison purposes.

Unit of analysis   The statistical focus of an analysis, which can be individuals, groups, or institutions, such as schools, churches, or entire communities.

Utilization research   Research on the structure and function of how research is used.

Variable   An attribute that allows the measurement of a construct of a theory.

Visitation metrics   Computer-generated statistics that help web site administrators analyze who is visiting their site, for how long, which features they are using most, and so forth.

Vulnerable populations   Groups who have greater susceptibility to poor health or social conditions or need greater protections, including prisoners, children, adolescents, the developmentally disabled, pregnant women, the elderly, minorities, immigrants, persons with mental, physical, or cognitive disabilities, and individuals who may not be able to make informed and free decisions about their participation in a research study and need special consideration and protection.

Web 2.0   Internet sites on which content is generated primarily by users receiving no or minimal payment, as opposed to professional Internet designers. These sites often facilitate interaction between users as a major part of their functionality.

Webmaster   A person who administers a web site and may also be the creator, editor, or owner of the site.

Web of Science   An electronic database covering more than 5,700 major journals across 164 scientific disciplines, including medicine and public health.

Windshield survey   A subjective assessment of a community taken while driving around and gathering impressions of activities, housing conditions, and resources such as schools, churches, and shops, as well as indications of potential problems such as the presence of vacant lots, trash, broken windows, or graffiti.

Working group   A formal or informal group of individuals working toward a specific goal or on a specific project.

YouTube   A social networking web site built around the uploading and sharing of videos.

REFERENCES

CHAPTER ONE

Bronfenbrenner, U. (1979). *The ecology of human development: Experiments by nature and design.* Cambridge, MA: Harvard University Press.

Central Intelligence Agency. (2008). *The 2008 world factbook.* Retrieved February 18, 2009, from www.cia .gov/library/publications/the-world-factbook.

Des Jarlais, D. C., Marmor, M., Paone, D., Titus, S., Shi, Q., Perlis, T., & Friedman, S. (1996). HIV incidence among injecting drug users in New York City syringe-exchange programmes. *Lancet, 348*(9033), 987–991.

Evans, L. (1990). Restraint effectiveness, occupant ejection from cars, and fatality reductions. *Accident Analysis and Prevention, 22*(2), 167–175.

Franco, E. L., Duarte-Franco, E., & Ferenczy, E. (2001). Cervical cancer: Epidemiology, prevention and the role of human papillomavirus infection. *Canadian Medical Association Journal, 164*(7), 1017–1025.

Grzywacz, J. G., & Fuqua, J. (2000). The social ecology of health: Leverage points and linkages. *Behavioral Medicine, 26*(3), 101–115.

Havens, D. H., & Zink, R. L. (1994). The "Back to Sleep" campaign. *Journal of Pediatric Health Care, 8*(5), 240–242.

Humphrey, L. L., Helfand, M., Chan, B. K., & Woolf, S. H. (2002). Breast cancer screening: A summary of the evidence for the U.S. Preventive Services Task Force. *Annals of Internal Medicine, 137*(5), 347–360.

James, J., Thomas, P., Cavan, D., & Kerr, D. (2004). Preventing childhood obesity by reducing consumption of carbonated drinks: Cluster randomised controlled trial. *British Medical Journal, 328*(7450), 1237–1241.

Mahler, H. (1981). The meaning of "health for all by the year 2000." *World Health Forum, 2*(1), 5–22.

McLeroy, K. R., Bibeau, D., Steckler, A., & Glanz, K. (1988). An ecological perspective on health promotion programs. *Health Education Quarterly, 15*(4), 351–377.

National Institute of Child Health and Human Development. (2008, October 16). *SIDS: "Back to Sleep" campaign.* Retrieved February 19, 2009, from www.nichd.nih.gov/sids.

Varghese, B., Maher, J. E., Peterman, T. A., Branson, B. M., & Steketee, R. W. (2002). Reducing the risk of sexual HIV transmission: Quantifying the per-act risk for HIV on the basis of choice of partner, sex act, and condom use. *Sexually Transmitted Diseases, 29*(1), 38–43.

Winzelberg, A. J., Classen, C., Alpers, G. W., Roberts, H., Koopman, C., Adams, R. E., Ernst, H., & Taylor, C. (2003). Evaluation of an Internet support group for women with primary breast cancer. *Cancer, 97*(5), 1164–1173.

CHAPTER TWO

Bernell, S. L., Mijanovich, T., & Weitzman, B. C. (2009). Does the racial composition of the school environment influence children's body mass index? *Journal of Adolescent Health, 45*(1), 40–46.

Browning, C. R., Leventhal, T., & Brooks-Gunn, J. (2004). Neighborhood context and racial differences in early adolescent sexual activity. *Demography, 41*(4), 697–720.

Collins, J. (2006). Addressing racial and ethnic disparities: Lessons from the REACH 2010 communities. *Journal of Health Care for the Poor and Underserved, 17*(Suppl. 2), 1–5.

Connell, J. P., Kubisch, A. C., Schorr, L. B., & Weiss, C. H. (Eds.). (1999). *New approaches to evaluating community initiatives.* Washington, DC: Aspen Institute.

Ennett, S.T., Faris, R., Hipp, J., Foshee, V. A., Bauman, K. E., Hussong, A., & Cai, L. (2008). Peer smoking, other peer attributes, and adolescent cigarette smoking: A social network analysis. *Prevention Science, 9*(2), 88–98.

Farquhar, J. W., Maccoby, N., Wood, P. D., Alexander, J. K., Breitrose, H., Brown, B. W., Haskell, W., McAlister, A., Meyer, A., Nash, J., & Stern, M. (1977). Community education for cardiovascular health. *Lancet, 1*(8023), 1192–1195.

Fishbein, M. (1996). Great expectations, or do we ask too much from community-level interventions? *American Journal of Public Health, 86*(8), 1075–1076.

Fortmann, S. P., Flora, J. A., Winkleby, M. A., Schooler, C. A., Taylor, C. B., & Farquhar, J. W. (1995). Community intervention trials: Reflections on the Stanford 5-City Project experience. *American Journal of Epidemiology, 142*(6), 576–586.

Fortmann, S. P., & Varady, A. N. (2000). Effects of a community-wide health education program on cardiovascular disease morbidity and mortality: The Stanford Five-City Project. *American Journal of Epidemiology, 152*(4), 316–323.

Freudenberg, N., Eng, E., Flay, B., Parcel, G., Rogers, T., & Wallerstein, N. (1994). Strengthening individual and community capacity to prevent disease and promote health: In search of relevant theories and principles. *Health Education and Behavior, 22*(3), 290–306.

Goodman, R. M., Steckler, A., Hoover, S., & Schwartz, R. (1993). A critique of contemporary community health promotion approaches based on a qualitative review of six programs in Maine. *American Journal of Health Promotion, 7*(3), 208–220.

Green, L. W., Wilson, A. L., & Lovato, C. Y. (1986). What changes can health promotion achieve and how long do these changes last? The trade-offs between expediency and durability. *Preventive Medicine, 15*(5), 508–521.

Howell, E. M., Pettit, K. L., Ormond, B. A., & Kingsley, G. T. (2003). Using the National Neighborhood Indicators Project to improve public health. *Journal of Public Health Management and Practice, 9*(3), 235–242.

Kok, G., Gottlieb, N. H., Commers, M., & Smerecnik, C. (2008). The ecological approach in health promotion programs: A decade later. *American Journal of Health Promotion, 22*(6), 437–442.

Merzel, C., & D'Afflitti, J. (2003). Reconsidering community-based health promotion: Promise, performance, and potential. *American Journal of Public Health, 93*(4), 557–574.

Minkler, M., & Wallerstein, N. (2003). *Community-based participatory research for health.* San Francisco: Jossey-Bass.

Mittelmark, M. B., Hunt, M. K., Heath, G. W., & Schmid, T. L. (1993). Realistic outcomes: Lessons from community-based research and demonstration programs for the prevention of cardiovascular diseases. *Journal of Public Health Policy,14*(4), 437–462.

Puska, P., Nissinen, A., Tuomilehto, J., Salonen, J. T., Koskela, K., McAlister, A., Kottke, T., Maccoby, N., & Farquhar, J. (1985). The community-based strategy to prevent coronary heart disease: Conclusions from the ten years of the North Karelia Project. *Annual Review of Public Health, 6,* 147–193.

Rose, G. (2001). Sick individuals and sick populations. *International Journal of Epidemiology, 30*(3), 427–432.

Thompson, B., Coronado, G., Snipes, S. A., & Puschel, K. (2003). Methodologic advances and ongoing challenges in designing community-based health promotion programs. *Annual Review of Public Health, 24,* 315–340.

Tosteson, A. N., Weinstein, M. C., Hunink, M. G., Mittleman, M. A., Williams, L. W., Goldman, P. A., & Goldman, L. (1997). Cost-effectiveness of populationwide educational approaches to reduce serum cholesterol levels. *Circulation, 95*(1), 24–30.

United States Department of Health and Human Services. (n.d.). *Planned Approach to Community Health: Guide for the local coordinator.* Retrieved February 17, 2009, from www.usmbha.org/Images/Projects/PromoVision/PATCH.pdf.

W. K. Kellogg Foundation. (2004, January). *Logic model development guide.* Retrieved February 17, 2009, from www.wkkf.org/Pubs/Tools/Evaluation/Pub3669.pdf.

CHAPTER THREE

Freis, E. D. (1967). Effects of treatment on morbidity in hypertension: Results in patients with diastolic blood pressures averaging 115 through 129 mm Hg. *Journal of the American Medical Association, 202*(11), 1028–1034.

Gostin, L. O. (2007). Biomedical research involving prisoners: Ethical values and legal regulation. *Journal of the American Medical Association, 297*(7), 737–740.

Hutt, L. E. (2003). Paying research subjects: Historical considerations. *Health Law Review, 12*(1), 16–21.

Jones, J. H. (1993). *Bad blood: The Tuskegee syphilis experiment.* New York: Free Press.

Mathews, C., Guttmacher, S., Coetzee, N., Magwaza, S., Stein, J., Lombard, C., Goldstein, S., & Coetzee, D. (2002). Evaluation of a video-based health education strategy to improve sexually transmitted disease partner notification in South Africa. *Sexually Transmitted Infections, 78*(1), 53–57.

Public Health Leadership Society. (2002). *Principles of the ethical practice of public health.* Retrieved February 20, 2009, from www.phls.org/home/section/3-26.

Tynan, M., Babb, S., & MacNeil, A. (2008). State smoking restrictions for private-sector worksites, restaurants, and bars: United States, 2004 and 2007. *Morbidity and Mortality Weekly Report, 57*(20), 549–552.

Weisstub, D. N., & Arboleda-Florez, J. (1997). Ethical research with the developmentally disabled. *Canadian Journal of Psychiatry, 42*(5), 492–496.

Wood, A., Grady, C., & Emanuel, E. J. (2002). *The crisis in human participants' research: Identifying the problems and proposing solutions.* Retrieved February 20, 2009, from www.bioethics.gov/background/emanuel paper.html.

CHAPTER FOUR

American Cancer Society. (2007). *Breast cancer facts and figures 2007–2008.* Retrieved February 26, 2009, from www.cancer.org/downloads/STT/BCFF-Final.pdf.

Anderson, J. V., Bybee, D. I., Brown, R. M., McLean, D. F., Garcia, E. M., Breer, M. L., & Schillo, B. A. (2001). 5 a day fruit and vegetable intervention improves consumption in a low-income population. *Journal of the American Dietetic Association, 101*(2), 195–202.

Centers for Disease Control and Prevention. (n.d.). *National breast and cervical cancer early detection program fact sheet, 2008–2009.* Retrieved February 26, 2009, from www.cdc.gov/cancer/nbccedp/bccpdfs/0809_nbccedp_fs.pdf.

Centers for Disease Control and Prevention. (1995). U.S. Public Health Service recommendations for human immunodeficiency virus counseling and voluntary testing to pregnant women. *Morbidity and Mortality Weekly Report, 44*(RR-7), 1–15.

Fowler, M. G., Lampe, M. A., Jamieson, D. J., Kourtis, A. P., & Rogers, M. F. (2007). Reducing the risk of mother-to-child human immunodeficiency virus transmission: Past successes, current progress and challenges, and future directions. *American Journal of Obstetrics & Gynecology, 197*(Suppl. 3), S3–S9.

Fuller, C. M., Galea, S., Caceres, W., Blaney, S., Sisco, S., & Vlahov, D. (2007). Multilevel community-based intervention to increase access to sterile syringes among injection drug users through pharmacy sales in New York City. *American Journal of Public Health,97*(1), 117–124.

Green, B. B., Cheadle, A., Pellegrini, A. S., & Harris, J. R. (2007). Active for life: A work-based physical activity program. *Preventing Chronic Disease, 4*(3), 1–7.

Kalichman, S. C., Rompa, D., & Cage, M. (2005). Group intervention to reduce HIV transmission risk behavior among persons living with HIV/AIDS. *Behavior Modification, 29*(2), 256–285.

Kalichman, S. C., Rompa, D., Cage, M., DiFonzo, K., Simpson, D., Austin, J., Luke, W., Buckles, J., Kyomugisha, F., Benotsch, E., Pinkerton, S., & Graham, J. (2001). Effectiveness of an intervention to reduce HIV transmission risks in HIV-positive people. *American Journal of Preventive Medicine, 21*(2), 84–92.

Kelly, G. A. (1955). *The psychology of personal constructs.* New York: Norton.

Lando, H. A., Pechacek, T. F., Pirie, P. L., Murray, D. M., Mittelmark, M. B., Lichtenstein, E., Nothwehr, F., & Gray, C. (1995). Changes in adult cigarette smoking in the Minnesota Heart Health Program. *American Journal of Public Health, 85*(2), 201–208.

McCaw, B., Berman, W. H., Syme, S. L., & Hunkeler, E. F. (2001). Beyond screening for domestic violence: A systems model approach in a managed care setting. *American Journal of Preventive Medicine, 21*(3), 170–176.

Mo-suwan, L., Pongprapai, S., Junjana, C., & Puetpaiboon, A. (1998). Effects of a controlled trial of a school-based exercise program on the obesity indexes of preschool children. *American Journal of Clinical Nutrition, 68*(5), 1006–1011.

Schoenwald, S., Brown, T., & Henggeler, S. (2000). Inside multisystemic therapy: Therapist, supervisory and program practices. *Journal of Emotional and Behavioral Disorders, 8*(2), 113–127.

Tabael, B. P., Burke, R., Constance, A., Hare, J., May-Aldrich, G., Parker, S. A., Scott, A., Stys, A., Chickering, J., & Herman, W. (2003). Community-based screening for diabetes in Michigan. *Diabetes Care, 26*(3), 668–670.

United States Department of Agriculture, Food and Nutrition Service. (2005). *Fit WIC: Programs to prevent childhood overweight in your community.* Retrieved February 26, 2009, from www.fns.usda.gov/oane/menu/published/WIC/FILES/fitwic.pdf.

Weatherill, S. A., Buxton, J. A., & Daly, P. C. (2004). Immunization programs in non-traditional settings. *Canadian Journal of Public Health, 95*(2), 133–137.

Winzelberg, A. J., Classen, C., Alpers, G. W., Roberts, H., Koopman, C., Adams, R. E., Ernst, H., Dev, P., & Taylor, C. (2003). Evaluation of an internet support group for women with primary breast cancer. *Cancer, 97*(5), 1164–1173.

CHAPTER FIVE

Abrar, S., Lovenduski, J., & Margetts, H. (2000). Feminist ideas and domestic violence policy change. *Political Studies, 48*(2), 239–262.

Bauermeister, J. A., Tross, S., & Ehrhardt, A. A. (2008). A review of HIV/AIDS system-level interventions. *AIDS and Behavior.* Retrieved February 27, 2009, from www.ncbi.nlm.nih.gov.

Beyer, J. M., & Trice, H. M. (1978). *Implementing change: Alcoholism policies in work organizations.* New York: Free Press.

Flores, A. L., Prue, C. E., & Daniel, K. L. (2007). Broadcasting behavior change: A comparison of the effectiveness of paid and unpaid media announcements to increase folic acid awareness, knowledge and consumption among Hispanic women of childbearing age. *Health Promotion Practice, 8*(2), 145–153.

Green, L. W., Ottoson, J. M., Garcia, C., & Hiatt, R. A. (2009). Diffusion theory and knowledge dissemination, utilization, and integration in public health. *Annual Review of Public Health.* Retrieved February 27, 2009, from www.ncbi.nlm.nih.gov.

Guidiotti, T. L., Ford, L., & Wheeler, M. (2000). The Fort McMurray Demonstration Project in social marketing: Theory, design, and evaluation. *American Journal of Preventive Medicine, 18*(2), 163–169.

Kelly, J. A., Somlai, A. M., Benotsch, E. G., Amirkhanian, Y. A., Fernandez, M. I., Stevenson, L. Y., Sitzler, C. A., McAuliffem, T. L., Brown, K. D., & Opgenorth, K. M. (2006). Programmes, resources, and needs of HIV-prevention nongovernmental organizations (NGOs) in Africa, Central/Eastern Europe and Central Asia, Latin America and the Caribbean. *AIDS Care, 18*(1), 12–21.

Kelly, J. A., Somlai, A. M., Benotsch, E .G., McAuliffe, T. L., Amirkhanian, Y. A., Brown, K. D., Stevenson, L. Y., Fernandez, M. I., Sitzler, C., Gore-Felton, C., Pinkerton, S. D., Weinhardt, L. S., & Opgenorth, K. M. (2004). Distance communication transfer of HIV prevention interventions to service providers. *Science, 305*(5692), 1953–1955.

Kelly, J. A., Somlai, A. M., DiFranceisco, W. J., Otto-Salaj, L. L., McAuliffe, T. L., Hackl, K. L., Heckman, T. G., Holtgrave, D. R., & Rompa, D. (2000). Bridging the gap between the science and service of HIV prevention: Transferring effective research-based HIV prevention interventions to community AIDS service providers. *American Journal of Public Health, 90*(7), 1082–1088.

Kotler, P. (1975). *Marketing for nonprofit organizations.* Englewood Cliffs, NJ: Prentice Hall.

Lewin, K. (1952). Group decision and social change. In G. E. Swanson, T. M. Newcomb, & E. L. Hartley (Eds.), *Readings in social psychology* (2nd ed., pp. 330–344). New York: Holt.

McAlister, A. L., Perry, C. L., & Parcel, G. S. (2008). How individuals, environments, and health behaviors interact: Social cognitive theory. In K. Glanz, B. K. Rimer, & K. Viswanath (Eds.), *Health behavior and health education: Theory, research, and practice* (4th ed., pp. 167–188). San Francisco: Jossey-Bass.

Prochaska, J. O., & DiClemente, C. C. (1983). Stages and processes of self-change of smoking: Towards an integrated model of change. *Journal of Consulting Clinical Psychology, 51,* 390–395.

Sabatier, P. A., & Jenkins-Smith, H. C. (Eds.). (1993). *Policy change and learning: An advocacy coalition approach.* Boulder, CO: Westview Press.

Smith, D. W., Steckler, A. B., McCormick, L. K., & McLeroy, K. R. (1995). Disseminating comprehensive school health curricula: Lessons learned from the North Carolina School Health and Tobacco Education Project. *Journal of Health Education, 26*(1), 37–43.

Weible, C. M., & Sabatier, P. A., & McQueen, K. (2009). Themes and variations: Taking stock of the advocacy coalition framework. *The Policy Studies Journal, 37*(1), 121–138.

Winkleby, M., Feighery, E., Altman, D., Kole, S., & Tencati, E. (2001). Engaging ethnically diverse teens in a substance use prevention advocacy program. *American Journal of Health Promotion, 15*(6), 433–436.

CHAPTER SIX

Creswell, J. W. (1998). *Qualitative inquiry and research design: Choosing among five traditions.* Thousand Oaks, CA: Sage.

Creswell, J. W., & Clark, V. L. (2007). *Designing and conducting mixed-methods research.* Thousand Oaks, CA: Sage.

Kelly, P. J., Ahmed, A., Martinez, E., & Peralez-Dieckmann, E. (2007). Cost analysis of obtaining post-intervention results in a cohort of high-risk adolescent girls. *Nursing Research, 56*(4), 269–274.

Lee, J. W., Jones, P. S., Mineyama, Y., & Zhang, X. E. (2002). Cultural differences in responses to a Likert scale. *Research in Nursing and Health, 25*(4), 295–306.

Lofland, J., & Lofland, L. (1995). *Analyzing social settings* (3rd ed.). Belmont, CA: Wadsworth.

Mirkin, R. M. (2005). *Statistics for the social sciences.* Thousand Oaks, CA: Sage.

Munro, B. (2005). *Statistical methods for health care research.* Philadelphia: Lippincott Williams & Wilkins.

Stommel, M., & Wills, C. (2003). *Clinical research: Concepts and principles for advanced practice nurses.* New York: Lippincott Williams & Wilkins.

CHAPTER SEVEN

Academy for Educational Development. (1994). Assessing and setting priorities for community needs. In *Handbook for HIV prevention community planning* (pp. 5-1–5-21). Washington, DC: Author.

Brownson, R. C., Baker, E. A., Leet, T. L., & Gillespie, K. N. (2003). *Evidence-based public health.* New York: Oxford University Press.

Gilmore, G. D., & Campbell, M. D. (2005). *Needs and capacity assessment strategies for health education and health promotion* (3rd ed.). Sudbury, MA: Jones and Bartlett.

Hanlon, J. J. (1973). Is there a future for local health departments? *Health Services Report, 88,* 898–901.

Hodges, B. C., & Videto, D. M. (2005). *Assessment and planning in health programs.* Sudbury, MA: Jones and Bartlett.

Kretzmann, J. P., & McKnight, J. L. (1993). *Building communities from the inside out: A path toward finding and mobilizing a community's assets.* Chicago: ACTA.

Petersen, D. J., & Alexander, G. R. (2001). *Needs assessment in public health: A practical guide for students and professionals.* New York: Kluwer Academic/Plenum.

Simons-Morton, B. G., Greene, W. H., & Gottlieb, N. H. (1995). *Introduction to health education and health promotion* (2nd ed.). Prospect Heights, IL: Waveland Press.

Soriano, F. I. (1995). *Conducting needs assessments: A multidisciplinary approach.* Thousand Oaks, CA: Sage.

Timmreck, T. C. (2003). *Planning, program development, and evaluation: A handbook for health promotion, aging, and health services* (2nd ed.). Sudbury, MA: Jones and Bartlett.

Van de Ven, A. H., & Delbecq, A. L. (1971). Nominal versus interacting groups for committee decision-making effectiveness. *Journal of the Academy of Management, 14*(2), 203–212.

Vilnius, D., & Dandoy, S. (1990). A priority rating system for public health programs. *Public Health Reports, 105*(5), 463–470.

Warren, R. B., & Warren, D. I. (1984). How to diagnose a neighborhood. In F. M. Cox, J. L. Erlich, J. Rothman, & J. E. Tropman (Eds.), *Tactics and techniques of community practice* (rev. ed., pp. 27–40). Itaska, IL: F. E. Peacock.

W. K. Kellogg Foundation. (2004, January). *Logic model development guide.* Retrieved February 17, 2009, from www.wkkf.org/Pubs/Tools/Evaluation/Pub3669.pdf.

CHAPTER EIGHT

Blank, K. (2007, November/December). Adolescents do what every day? *Substance Abuse and Mental Health Association Services Administration News, 15*(6). Retrieved February 27, 2009, from www.samhsa.gov/SAMHSA_News/VolumeXV_6/article12.htm.

Centers for Disease Control and Prevention. (1994a). Guidelines for school health programs to prevent tobacco use and addiction. *Morbidity and Mortality Weekly Report, 43*(RR-2), 1–18.

Centers for Disease Control and Prevention. (1994b). Preventing tobacco use among young people: A report of the Surgeon General—executive summary. *Morbidity and Mortality Weekly Report, 43*(RR-4), 1–10.

Centers for Disease Control and Prevention. (2008, December). *Logic model basics.* Retrieved February 27, 2009, from www.cdc.gov/HealthyYouth/evaluation/pdf/brief2.pdf.

Centers for Disease Control and Prevention. (2009, January 29). *Tobacco use: Targeting the nation's leading killer.* Retrieved February 27, 2009, from www.cdc.gov/NCCDPHP/publications/aag/osh.htm.

Centers for Disease Control and Prevention. (n.d.). *Evaluation guide: Writing SMART objectives.* Retrieved February 27, 2009, from www.cdc.gov/dhdsp/state_program/evaluation_guides/smart_objectives.htm.

DiFranza, J. R. (1992). Preventing teenage tobacco addiction. *Journal of Family Practice, 34*(6), 753–756.

Flores, R. (1995). Dance for health: Improving fitness in African American and Hispanic adolescents. *Public Health Reports, 110*(2), 189–193.

Friis, R. H., & Sellers, T. A. (2004). *Epidemiology for public health practice* (3rd ed.). Sudbury, MA: Jones and Bartlett.

Jason, L. A., Ji, P. Y., Anes, M. D., & Birkhead, S. H. (1991). Active enforcement of cigarette control laws in the prevention of cigarette sales to minors. *Journal of the American Medical Association, 266*(22), 3159–3161.

Kaplan, S. A., & Garrett, K. E. (2005). The use of logic models by community-based initiatives. *Evaluation and Program Planning, 28*(2), 167–172.

Keay, K. D., Woodruff, S. I., Wildey, M. B., & Kenney, E. M. (1993). Effect of a retailer intervention on cigarette sales to minors in San Diego County, California. *Tobacco Control, 2,* 145–151.

Luepker, R. V., Johnson, C. A., Murray, D. M., & Pechacek, T. F. (1983). Prevention of cigarette smoking: Three-year follow-up of an education program for youth. *Journal of Behavioral Medicine, 6*(1), 53–62.

Manlove, J. (1998). The influence of high school dropout and school disengagement on the risk of school-age pregnancy. *Journal of Research on Adolescence, 8*(2), 187–220.

McCawley, P. F. (n.d.). *The logic model for program planning and evaluation.* Retrieved February 27, 2009, from www.uidaho.edu/extension/LogicModel.pdf.

Mensch, B., & Kandel, D. B. (1992). Drug use as a risk factor for premarital teen pregnancy and abortion in a national sample of young white women. *Demography, 29*(3), 409–429.

Miller, K. E., Sabo, D. F., Farrell, M. P., Barnes, G. M., & Melnick, M. J. (1998). Athletic participation and sexual behavior in adolescents: The different worlds of boys and girls. *Journal of Health and Social Behavior, 39*(2), 108–123.

Murphy, M., Nevill, A., Neville, C., Biddle, S., & Hardman, A. (2002). Accumulating brisk walking for fitness, cardiovascular risk, and psychological health. *Medicine & Science in Sports & Exercise, 34*(9), 1468–1474.

Newton, R. A. (2006). Prevention of falls at home: Home hazard and safety assessment and management. *Annals of Long-Term Care: Clinical Care and Aging, 14*(11), 28–33.

Nilsson, M., Stenlund, H., Bergström, E., Weinehall, L., & Janlert, U. (2006). It takes two: Reducing adolescent smoking uptake through sustainable adolescent-adult partnership. *Journal of Adolescent Health, 39*(6), 880–886.

O'Connor, C., Small, S. A., & Cooney, S. M. (2007). Culturally appropriate prevention programming: What do we know about evidence-based programs for culturally and ethnically diverse youth and their families? *What Works: Wisconsin Research to Practice Series, 1.* Retrieved February 27, 2009, from www.uwex.edu/ces/flp/families/whatworks_01.pdf.

Pentz, M. A., MacKinnon, D. P., Flay, B. R., Hansen, W. B., Johnson, C. A., & Dwyer, J. H. (1989). Primary prevention of chronic diseases in adolescence: Effects of the Midwestern Prevention Project on tobacco use. *American Journal of Epidemiology, 130*(4), 713–724.

Spoth, R. L., Randall, G. K., Trudeau, L., Shin, C., & Redmond, C. (2008). Substance use outcomes 5-1/2 years past baseline for partnership-based, family-school preventive interventions. *Drug and Alcohol Dependence, 96*(1–2), 57–68.

Stanton, W. R., Mahalski, P. A., McGee, R., & Silva, P. A. (1993). Reasons for smoking or not smoking in early adolescence. *Addictive Behaviors, 18*(3), 321–329.

Stead, L. F., & Lancaster, T. (2000). Interventions for preventing tobacco sales to minors. *Tobacco Control, 9,* 169–176.

Taylor-Powell, E. (1999). Evaluating collaboratives: Challenges and practice. *The Evaluation Exchange, 5*(2/3), 6–7.

Taylor-Powell, E., Jones, L., & Henert, E. (2002). *Enhancing program performance with logic models.* Retrieved February 27, 2009, from www.uwex.edu/ces/lmcourse.

W. K. Kellogg Foundation. (2004, January). *Logic model development guide.* Retrieved February 17, 2009, from www.wkkf.org/Pubs/Tools/Evaluation/Pub3669.pdf.

Wakefield, M. A., Chaloupka, F. J., Kaufman, N. J., Orleans, C. T., Barker, D. C., & Ruel, F. E. (2000). Effect of restrictions on smoking at home, at school, and in public places on teenage smoking: Cross-sectional study. *British Medical Journal, 321*(7257), 333–337.

Walter, H. J., Vaugh, R. D., & Wynder, E. L. (1989). Primary prevention of cancer among children: Changes in cigarette smoking and diet after six years of intervention. *Journal of the National Cancer Institute, 81*(13), 995–997.

Wildey, M., Woodruff, S., Argo, A., Keay, K., Kenney, E., & Conway, T. (1995). Sustained effects of educating retailers to reduce cigarette sales to minors. *Public Health Reports, 110,* 625–629.

Woodruff, S. I., Erickson, A. D., Wildey, M. B., & Kenney, E. M. (1993). Changing retailer knowledge, attitudes, and behaviors related to cigarette sales to minors. *Journal of Community Psychology, 21,* 234–245.

CHAPTER TEN

Kirkpatrick, D., & Kirkpatrick, J. (2006). *Implementing the four levels: A practical guide for effective evaluation of training programs.* San Francisco: Berrett Koehler.

Shadish, W., Cook, T., & Campbell, D. (2002). *Experimental and quasi-experimental designs for generalized causal inference.* Boston: Houghton Mifflin.

CHAPTER ELEVEN

Brown, L., & Brown, M. (2001). *Demystifying grant seeking.* San Francisco: Jossey-Bass.

Browning, B. (2008). *Grant writing for dummies* (4th ed.). New York: Wiley.

Carlson, M. (2002). *Winning grants step by step.* San Francisco: Jossey-Bass.

Foundation Center. (2009). Frequently asked questions. Retrieved March 10, 2009, from http://foundationcenter.org/getstarted/faqs.

Karsh, E., & Fox, A. (2003). *The only grant writing book you'll ever need.* New York: Carroll & Graf.

Scheirer, M. (2005). Is sustainability possible? A review and commentary on empirical studies of program sustainability. *American Journal of Evaluation, 26,* 320–347.

CHAPTER THIRTEEN

Masi, C. M., Suarez-Balcazar, Y., Cassey, M. Z., Kinney, L., & Plotrowski, Z. H. (2003). Internet access and empowerment: A community-based health initiative. *Journal of General Internal Medicine, 18,* 525–530.

Thompson, D., Baranowski, T., Cullen, K., Watson, K., Liu, Y., Canada, A., Bhatt, R., & Zakeri, I. (2008). Food, fun, and fitness internet program for girls: Pilot evaluation of an e-health youth obesity prevention program examining predictors of obesity. *Preventive Medicine, 47,* 494–497.

Ybarra, M. L., & Bull, S. S. (2007). Current trends in internet- and cell phone–based HIV prevention and intervention programs. *Current HIV/AIDS Reports, 4,* 201–207.

Zrebiac, J. F. (2005). Internet communities: Do they improve coping with diabetes? *The Diabetes Educator, 31,* 825–832.

INDEX

Page references followed by *fig* indicate an illustrated figure; followed by *t* indicate a table.

CPSIA information can be obtained
at www.ICGtesting.com
Printed in the USA
BVHW02n2116230118
505798BV00005B/6/P